Praise for *Power Up Your Brain*

"Dr. Perlmutter and Dr. Villoldo bring together the long-separated disciplines of science and spirituality to help us gain access to the parts of the brain that define us as human beings. This book applies leading-edge science to our quest for enlightenment and gives us practical tools, including specific dietary and lifestyle recommendations, to improve our well-being."

— **Andrew Weil, M.D.,** author of
8 Weeks to Optimum Health and *Healthy Aging*

"The shaman and physician for millennia were the same person until the 19th century when they were split apart in the name of science. Now through the lens of 21st-century science, Villoldo and Perlmutter bring them back together, illuminating the web that links together our physical and metaphysical energy. For anyone feeling a loss of energy of body or soul, **Power Up Your Brain** *is your guide to restoration and rejuvenation of your deepest energies."*

— **Mark Hyman, M.D.,** *New York Times* best-selling author of
The UltraMind Solution

"This is the book we've been waiting for! With leading-edge information that's easy to understand, Alberto Villoldo and David Perlmutter have masterfully woven 21st-century science with the indigenous wisdom of the past to reveal the 'missing link' in the modern story of life—the role of our brain's health in the quality of our spiritual experience. In doing so they offer us a practical wisdom that we can use to empower our lives immediately! This book is a must for anyone seriously interested in moving beyond the conventional ideas of what enlightenment is and how to achieve it."

— **Gregg Braden,** *New York Times* best-selling author of
The Divine Matrix and *Fractal Time*

POWER
UP YOUR BRAIN

Also by David Perlmutter

RAISE A SMARTER CHILD BY KINDERGARTEN:
Build a Better Brain and Increase IQ by up to 30 Points
(with Carol Colman)

THE BETTER BRAIN BOOK:
The Best Tools for Improving Memory, Sharpness, and Preventing
Aging of the Brain (with Carol Colman)

BRAINRECOVERY.COM:
Powerful Therapy for Challenging Brain Disorders

LIFEGUIDE: Your Guide to a Longer and Healthier Life

Also by Alberto Villoldo

*ILLUMINATION: The Shaman's Way of Healing**

COURAGEOUS DREAMING:
*How Shamans Dream the World into Being**

*YOGA, POWER, AND SPIRIT: Patanjali the Shaman**

THE FOUR INSIGHTS:
*Wisdom, Power, and Grace of the Earthkeepers**

MENDING THE PAST AND HEALING THE FUTURE WITH
*SOUL RETRIEVAL**

SHAMAN, HEALER, SAGE: How to Heal Yourself
and Others with the Energy Medicine of the Americas

DANCE OF THE FOUR WINDS:
Secrets of the Inca Medicine Wheel (with Erik Jendresen)

ISLAND OF THE SUN: Mastering the Inca Medicine Wheel
(with Erik Jendresen)

*Available from Hay House

Please visit:
Hay House USA: **www.hayhouse.com®**
Hay House Australia: **www.hayhouse.com.au**
Hay House UK: **www.hayhouse.co.uk**
Hay House South Africa: **www.hayhouse.co.za**
Hay House India: **www.hayhouse.co.in**

Published and distributed in the United States by: Hay House, Inc.: www.hayhouse.com • *Published and distributed in Australia by:* Hay House Australia Pty. Ltd.: www.hayhouse.com.au • *Published and distributed in the United Kingdom by:* Hay House UK, Ltd.: www.hayhouse.co.uk • *Published and distributed in the Republic of South Africa by:* Hay House SA (Pty), Ltd.: www.hayhouse.co.za • *Distributed in Canada by:* Raincoast: www.raincoast.com • *Published in India by:* Hay House Publishers India: www.hayhouse.co.in

Design: Riann Bender

Page 105: Image reprinted from *The Lancet,* Vol. 358, Annachiara Cagnin, et al, "In-vivo measurement of activated microglia in dementia," page 465, 2001 ©, with permission from Elsevier.

Library of Congress Cataloging-in-Publication Data

Perlmutter, David, M.D.
  Power up your brain : the neuroscience of enlightenment / David Perlmutter and Alberto Villoldo. -- 1st ed.
    p. ; cm.
  Includes bibliographical references.
  ISBN 978-1-4019-2817-9 (hardcover : alk. paper) 1. Mental healing.
2. Neurosciences. 3. Shamanism. 4. Enlightenment.
I. Villoldo, Alberto. II. Title.
  [DNLM: 1. Spiritual Therapies. 2. Neurosciences. 3. Shamanism. WB 885]
  RZ400.P46 2011
  615.8'51--dc22
                              2010029233

Hardcover ISBN: 978-1-4019-2817-9
Digital ISBN: 978-1-4019-3084-4

14 13 12 11   4 3 2 1
1st edition, February 2011

Printed in the United States of America

POWER
UP YOUR BRAIN

*The Neuroscience
of Enlightenment*

**DAVID PERLMUTTER,
M.D., F.A.C.N.**

ALBERTO VILLOLDO, PH.D.

HAY HOUSE, INC.
Carlsbad, California • New York City
London • Sydney • Johannesburg
Vancouver • Hong Kong • New Delhi

To our wives, Marcela Lobos and Leize Perlmutter—
ever supportive, loving, and understanding partners.

CONTENTS

PUBLISHER'S FOREWORD

Shamanism and neuroscience: what do they have in common? They are both keys to personal health and wellness, mental excellence, spiritual awareness, growth and prosperity, improved personal relationships, a higher quality of life, and a greater ability to perform and contribute to society—to name a few benefits.

Yet, seldom have we seen these words—*shamanism* and *neuroscience*—used in the same sentence. Why is that? Because we have been living in a time of reductionism during which the realm of spirit and the domain of science have been separated, split, divided, and divorced from one another.

This was not always so. For millennia, shamans were also astronomers, wizards were scientists, spiritual seekers were explorers, and researchers were risk takers. Their opinions were valued by emperors, chieftains, tsars, kings, and potentates. That is, until the time when established authorities—the popes and princes of the powerful status quo—labeled visionaries as heretics and decreed that religion and science should follow their disparate paths.

Fortunately, the relationship of spirit and matter, while subjugated to the background, was never totally erased from human consciousness. Scientists have always suspected that a connection, preserved in some basal paradigm, exists between the soul and the brain. And this thought began to reemerge a few decades ago, phrased as the mind-body-spirit connection.

And now two men, two seers—a shaman and a scientist—are combining their experiences and expertise to explore the totality that includes all of the spirit world and all of the scientific world—as One.

Power Up Your Brain: The Neuroscience of Enlightenment is a collaboration of Dr. David Perlmutter, a neuroscientist and practicing neurologist; and Dr. Alberto Villoldo, a medical anthropologist and shaman. Unlike the majority of scientists who have investigated meditation and the extraordinary feats of yogis, both of them are hands-on clinicians, helping countless patients heal their emotions, repair their brains, and enlighten their minds. Therefore, this book's message is a reunion of ethereal spirit and hard science. And its content is a spiritual blessing and a physical benefit to you—and to others with whom you share this story.

Why? Because *Power Up Your Brain* is blend of deep shamanic truths and profound scientific facts.

Do David Perlmutter and Alberto Villoldo dare to use the words *neuroscience* and *shamanism* in the same sentence? Yes! Resoundingly, yes. Because, in effect, neuroscience and shamanism are cut from the same cloth, threads in the same fabric of human history and human evolution.

PREFACE

David Perlmutter:
Explorations, Then and Now

As we followed the shaman up the mountain along the ancient stone pathway crafted by the Inca some six centuries ago, the silence was broken only by the sound of his flute. Our destination was Ollantaytambo, near Machu Picchu, not only one of Peru's best-preserved archaeological sites but also a site of great spiritual significance.

My companions seemed to be energized by their spirited endeavor, yet I was more concerned with the pounding in my head. The shock to my body of traveling quickly, from sea level in Florida to almost 10,000 feet in the Andes, focused my attention on the inescapable fact that I was suffering from shortness of breath and blurred vision. Thankfully, my wife and two children seemed less affected.

One of the shamans traveling with us noticed my distress and offered me a handful of coca leaves to chew. I decided to try it instead of the acetazolamide I carried in my backpack in case of high-altitude sickness. Soon I felt numbness in my mouth and, very quickly, my symptoms disappeared!

How did this descendant of the Inca know that the leaves of the *Erythroxylum coca* plant could help with the symptoms of high-altitude sickness? The obvious answer is that it was the benefit of ancient wisdom, yet that only partially satisfied me. It seemed improbable that some hapless forebear had been chosen to chew his way through all the local plants to check their medicinal use. Meanwhile, my companion studied my countenance, much as I would observe my own patients. Meeting his gaze, I realized that his knowledge of the coca leaf did not come from lessons learned but was rooted in a profound knowledge of soul and spirit—not a concept that sat easily with my Western medical training, and yet I felt moved to accept it.

My journey to the Andes in the company of my family was inspired by my wife after she had read several books by Dr. Alberto Villoldo. We chose this expedition *because* Alberto was leading it, and it was not long after my healing encounter that I had a chance to speak with him. Our conversation flowed naturally, without elaborate introductions, and soon revolved around a discussion of the sustainability of cultures living seemingly off the grid. Later that same day, back at our hotel, I asked Alberto about the shaman's apparently unique ability to access complex information by means of intuition.

"That has been my mission for the past thirty years," Alberto replied, explaining that he had made it his life's work to discover how such unassuming individuals are able to amass such a vast compendium of information. "It is not knowledge that comes from others," he continued. "It comes from the source of all knowledge, which is the Great Spirit. The sages are able to tap into this wisdom, and to a certain extent we all have the potential to do this, not just indigenous peoples. After all, there have been individuals throughout the ages and in all cultures who were considered enlightened."

I returned to my medical practice serving patients with a variety of challenging brain disorders, my treatment plans always integrating lifestyle issues and nutritional interventions with standard pharmaceutical-based approaches. This less than traditional neurological methodology allowed me to gain a deep understanding of health issues while retaining a mind-set that was open to new ideas. Nevertheless, I continued to be challenged by patients who suffered diseases that were well beyond the scope of neurology alone, including cancer, advanced arthritis, diabetes, and other equally challenging disorders.

I began to focus on the small but growing number of patients who were actually able to regain their health despite what could have been a diagnosis of incurable disease. What was it about these patients that turned things around? The answer was presented to me late one Friday afternoon during a consultation with a woman suffering from chronic progressive multiple sclerosis, a frequently fatal and crippling auto-immune brain disorder.

We had placed Beth on our standard array of nutritional supplements, specific essential fatty acids, and nutrient injections for the disorder several years before. Although her decline had slowed somewhat, she was forced to use a walker and even a wheelchair at times. That afternoon, however, my staff and I were astounded to see her walking down our hallway unassisted.

"We are putting you on our miracle list," I told her, referring to the growing number of our patients whose improvements could not be explained by medical science.

In the examining room, we explored what had changed in her life and to what she attributed her miraculous improvement.

"I have been studying shamanism for a few years," she replied, scrutinizing my face for any sign of familiarity with the term. "Basically, I've gained the ability to tap into what I call *healing energy*," Beth continued. "Not only am I doing so much better as far as my MS is concerned, but I also feel really peaceful and positive about my life. I've been practicing some meditation techniques for years," she explained, "but they never really clicked until about three months ago."

Over the coming months, I began to notice that we were putting more and more people on the miracle list. And it was becoming clear to me that, overwhelmingly, the patients who achieved the most profound recoveries were those engaged in some form of meditative or spiritual practice. Whether they repeated affirmations, meditated, or prayed in some fashion, virtually all of these patients were somehow connecting with what the shaman had referred to as the Great Spirit.

There were several other characteristics in the lifestyles of our miracle-list patients that began to stand out in addition to their spiritual practices. Many of them had adopted the practice of fasting from time to time. Almost all of them engaged in some form of physical exercise. And an overwhelming number were taking some form of docosahexaenoic acid (DHA). The use of this omega-3 supplement was no doubt the result of my personal enthusiasm for it; indeed, I later discovered that it has a special attribute that was probably playing a much larger role in enhancing the efficacy of lifestyle changes in my patients than I had previously imagined.

Over the next three years, my encounters with Alberto evolved into a close friendship, and we realized that we should put our heads together and collaborate. For it had become clear to us that access to the Great Spirit or Divine Energy—that natural force which is called by so many names—is available to all. In a sense, we are all shamans, and the most advanced teachings in cellular biology are validating lifestyle activities that, for centuries, have been paving the way to enlightenment through meditative practices not just for the chosen few but for all who care to learn. Our collaboration explores the implications of this not only for individuals but for all of humanity.

■ ■ ■

Alberto Villoldo:
Journey from the Brain Laboratory to Enlightenment

Over time, I grew accustomed to the stench of formaldehyde. Stinky five-gallon vats held all kinds of brains—sheep brains, cow brains, human brains—but it was the only laboratory space I was able to wrangle from the biology department at San Francisco State University. And so, under these conditions, surrounded by hundreds of brains, I conducted my research into how the mind creates psychosomatic health or disease and how shamans are able to cure illness.

One day, two years into my research, I realized that I had been viewing the mind through the wrong lens. I had been trying to understand a spiritual tradition of indigenous America by looking at changes in brain and blood chemistry. The following week, I resigned my post at the university and shut down my lab. And before the month was over, I had purchased a one-way ticket to the Peruvian Amazon to study the shamans in their own environment. My best friend, a medical student, gave me a very large hunting knife as a gift, with a note that said, "You might need this in the Upper Amazon." Everyone I knew, including my own family, thought I was mad to throw away a promising career in academia to follow a harebrained dream of being an explorer and adventurer. I had my own doubts and reservations, but I shared them with no one. I was a city boy who had never set foot in the jungle. But I was sure of one thing: I would not find answers about the mind in a laboratory.

I spent the next quarter of a century traveling and studying with the most renowned sages of the Americas. During that time, I witnessed extraordinary cures—persons whom Western medicine would have long given up on returned to health through ways I could only ascribe to a miracle or spontaneous remission. Over time, I became an apprentice to the shamans and learned their healing practices and methodologies. Yet part of me always felt like an outsider. One old Indian I worked with for many years, a man who eventually became my mentor, explained to me: "That's because your God is a descending God. He comes down from the heavens on rare occasions to touch those of us here on the Earth; whereas our deity is an ascending divinity who rises from the Earth like the golden corn and resides among us. Our creative force is known as Pachamama, the Divine Mother."

The sages I studied with worked with the Divine Mother, an energy or intelligence they were capable of interacting with to heal their patients. They believed that we ourselves *are* this divine energy embodied in matter, much like ribbons of sunlight that wrap themselves around the trunks of trees and then release their light when we place a log into the fire. They claimed they were able to *see* emanations of this energy around the body of a person in the form of a luminous matrix. Dark spots in the matrix indicate the presence of disease, they said, even if the illness had not yet manifested in the physical body.

After many years, I also learned to *sense* this luminous field and to comprehend the shamans' concept of all life being interconnected through strands of light. In the beginning, my scientific mind had to grasp this notion by explaining to myself that we eat animals that eat grasses that feed on sunlight. I reminded myself that chlorophyll turns light into carbohydrates, such as wheat and other grains, and that we turn carbohydrates back into light inside our cells for fuel through a process known as the Krebs Cycle. With time, my logical brain relaxed its vise-like grip on my awareness, and I was able to perceive more directly the luminous weave of all creation.

With time, I learned that trauma leaves an almost indelible signature that a healer can perceive in her clients' luminous field. Healers believe that this marks a person's experience of health or disease for their entire life, like a cross that each of us has to shoulder. A shaman can help people to lighten their load, perhaps even help them understand the lessons they needed to learn from the original trauma they experienced, but it is up to each person to choose whether they carry their cross lightly, discard it altogether, or become burdened and overwhelmed beneath the weight. According to the shamans, the way to clear these marks and shed this burden that defines our personality and our health is by healing our toxic emotions via energy medicine.

I learned the practice of energy medicine during my years with the shamans and now teach it to students in the United States and Europe. Our graduates learn to use timeless healing techniques to help friends, family members, and clients. As modern shamans, we also know that if a person wants to be healed of disease and be truly free and enlightened, then it is essential to strengthen the feminine life force within. This requires fasting, prayer, and meditation, combined with the use of healing herbs and plants.

During my years studying with the shamans, I learned about their belief in the Divine Mother, which we each have the potential to discover in nature. This was not the bearded old man whose image I had come to associate with "God." Rather, this was a force that infused all of creation, a sea of energy and consciousness that we all swim in and are part of. I came to understand that our Western notions of the divine are perhaps a masculine version of this life force that infuses every cell in our bodies, that animates all living beings, and that even fuels stars. The shamans helped me to develop an original and fulfilling relationship with the power of Pachamama.

In 2006, on one of my yearly expeditions to the Andes, I met David Perlmutter. He first caught my attention as we were hiking up the ancient Inca stone steps to reach the Temple of the Winds, near the village of Ollantaytambo. He was short of breath but was greatly helped by chewing the coca leaves that the local people consider medicinal. His pace and demeanor picked up, and later we struck up a comfortable and easy conversation, as if we had always known each other.

I had heard of David and his work over the years and was delighted to hear he was also interested in indigenous healing practices. As we talked on that first day of our encounter, I mentioned the shamans' notion of how important it is to restore the feminine life force, and his face immediately lit up. "Yes," he remarked, "it's the mitochondria."

On hearing this, I nearly fell off my chair. Here was the link between the ancient shamanic practices and modern neuroscience. I remembered that our mitochondria are inherited only from our mother's lineage. Here was the source, inside each cell of every living creature, of the feminine life force that sages speak about. I became very excited when he mentioned how these energy factories seemed to be breaking down under the continual barrage of stress in our fast-paced lives and from biochemical toxins, including mercury, pesticides, and water and air pollution. David hinted that the ancient shamanic practices, including prayer, fasting, and meditation as well as dietary supplementation with special herbs, help restore mitochondrial function.

The more we conversed, the more obvious it became to both of us that there are many elements of *ancient* healing and spiritual practices that can be described in *modern* neurological terms. The feminine life force of Pachamama could be found in our mitochondria; the marks of trauma in our Luminous Energy Field correspond to neural networks in the brain that produce toxic emotions and define our personality.

I was overjoyed. Here was the missing element that had eluded me in the Amazon but that had been all around me during my days at the laboratory, ensconced between shelves stacked with chemically preserved brains.

The fact is that, although I had succeeded in translating ancient shamanic healing methods into scientifically sound practices and my students at the Healing the Light Body School and patients reported extraordinary life transformations, some found it very difficult to break free from their destructive beliefs and emotions. It was also impractical for my students to do what I had done during 25 years in the Amazon and Andes; namely, to fast for many days in the wilderness while eating only special barks and berries.

David had knowledge of rich brain nutrients that could accomplish the same thing—perhaps even more finely and certainly more conveniently than the rigorous diets the shamans prescribed. He understood how to repair the mitochondria and restore the feminine life force. He knew how to prime the brain for enlightenment. I, meanwhile, had studied in depth the shamanic and yogic practices that would help to switch on the higher-order functions of our brain to help it heal from trauma and experience joy.

What if we could bring these methodologies together to help our students and patients heal their brain, restore their health, and experience freedom from destructive emotions like anger and fear?

INTRODUCTION

Enlightenment. This elusive state has been the focus of some of the greatest minds throughout history. Thousands of people have dedicated their lives to its pursuit. We see images of monks sitting peacefully on meditation cushions . . . nuns kneeling in prayer . . . shamans living in the wilds of the Amazon. And while these representations of enlightened individuals may be accurate, they also imply that this desired state is reserved for a privileged few.

We believe, however, that enlightenment is available to all those who are willing to dedicate the time and effort necessary to attain it. Finding this state does not require a lifestyle that is incompatible with surviving in the modern Western world. And the rewards of enlightenment are not limited to the attainment of spiritual knowledge enjoyed by the contemplative mystic. They can also be reaped in the discovery of DNA sequencing by the innovative scientist, the preparation of a mouth-watering meal by the inventive chef, or the creation of an inspiring masterpiece by the insightful artist. We believe that enlightenment promises everyone the possibility for innovation, extraordinary creativity, and inner peace.

We also believe that the search for enlightenment can be accelerated by following a practice focused on awakening the power of the higher brain. When our higher brain functions are engaged, we have the potential to change our lives both spiritually and biologically.

But to achieve this desired state of consciousness, we must not only master ancient enlightenment techniques but also restore the brain's health at the cellular level. These two goals are inextricably linked.

YOUR OPTIMAL BRAIN

Anger, fear, jealousy, greed, and worry, while commonplace, undermine our inner peace and sense of self-worth. But even on a weekend meditation retreat or during a walk in the quiet and stillness of the woods, the mind continues to chase thoughts, compose to-do lists, and fret about activities not yet completed and situations not yet resolved. Hard as we might try to sit quietly and empty our mind of thoughts, it continues to gravitate toward the unfinished business of our past.

Power Up Your Brain helps you understand why, instead of operating at its optimal level of functioning, your brain instead relies on the neural networks created by the prehistoric, survival-at-all-costs brain regions—the reptilian brain and the limbic brain. It also shows you how to overcome the toxic emotions of your old wiring, the conditioning based on negative experiences from the past. By healing that prehistoric brain, you engage newer, higher, more evolved brain structures—the neocortex and, specifically, the prefrontal cortex—which will help you eliminate fear, poverty mentality, and anger from your life. This is done through the creation of new neural networks in your brain.

Until quite recently, most brain researchers held that, even though the brain is malleable in the early years of a child's development, the window of opportunity for changing its wiring slams shut by around the age of seven years. While it is true that the brain of a fetus or a young child is like a dry sponge, with the potential to soak up all the knowledge, beliefs, and behaviors it needs to survive in its new worldly environment, the premise that the brain can no longer be rewired past a certain early age has now been upended.

Leading-edge neuroscience research now confirms that we can grow new brain cells and change the actual networks in the brain. Once we provide our neurons with specific nutrients lacking in our everyday diet and embark on stimulating new activities, we can establish new neural networks that help transform limiting beliefs and behaviors and recapture long-lost feelings of joy, optimism, and tranquility.

To achieve these benefits, you must start by learning how the brain functions and how your mitochondria have become compromised.

A HEALTHY BODY

In the language of neuroscience, enlightenment is the condition of optimal mitochondrial and brain functioning that allows us to experience both well-being and inner peace *and* the urge to create and innovate. Mitochondria are the energy factories at work within your cells. They impact your moods, your vitality, your aging process, and even how you might die. They are also in charge of the elimination of old cells and replacement with new cells, a function that occurs automatically, without your conscious awareness.

The mitochondria are influenced by the foods you eat, the amount of calories you ingest, the extent to which you exercise your body, and the inclusion of specific nutrients.

Power Up Your Brain will give you access to keys encoded in your mitochondrial DNA that, until now, have been password-protected due to an inability to reverse the damage caused by free-radical damage to the brain. When you unlock this code, you break free of the illness-ridden journey that many Westerners suffer from cradle to grave. With your mitochondria restored, your cells will be able to express the genes that promote brain health and physical longevity, and you won't have to continue perpetuating the ills and traumas of your family of origin.

THE POWER UP YOUR BRAIN PROGRAM

Blue Zones are regions on the planet where ten times more people reach the age of 100 compared with people in the United States. Dan Buettner, a *National Geographic* writer and researcher, wrote a book about this phenomenon and reported that these individuals have certain traits in common, including calorie reduction (they eat 25 percent less than what you would need to feel full), avoiding meat and processed foods, and living lives that have meaning and purpose.[1] Buettner cites a Danish scientific study of twins that indicates that genes dictate less than 25 percent of a person's health and longevity. The remaining 75 percent is determined by lifestyle factors: what you eat, how you love and are loved, how much you exercise, and how you discover meaning in your life.

Lifestyle factors actually modify our genetic expression by shutting off the genes that predispose us to malignancy and disease. Our mitochondria regulate the switching on or off of these genes. Therefore, to live long and live well, we need optimally functioning mitochondria.

At our facilities—the Center for Energy Medicine in Los Lobos, Chile, and the Perlmutter Health Center in Naples, Florida—we help our clients restore their mitochondria to repair their brains. Our protocols utilize intravenous glutathione and hyperbaric oxygen to optimize mitochondrial function as well as foods and supplements that help undo the damage done to the brain by years of stressful living. We find that mitochondria, the mind, and the brain respond extraordinarily quickly to these interventions. Then, through shamanic meditation practices, we can heal from toxic emotions and discover inner peace.

But you do not have to take part in one of our seven-day intensives to accomplish this. In *Power Up Your Brain*, we present a program to help you do the same things: heal your mitochondria and rewire your brain for peace and joy instead of suffering. We combine two complementary strategies: brain-specific nutrients used in conjunction with fasting and enlightenment practices. The neuronutrients recommended by Dr. Perlmutter work to repair regions in your brain that have been affected by stress, psychological trauma, and degenerative brain disease to help grow new brain cells and turn on the genes responsible for longevity, improved immunity, and enhanced brain function. And the enlightenment practices pioneered by Alberto Villoldo, Ph.D., help awaken brain regions that allow peace, compassion, innovation, and joy to arise naturally. Together, they will enable you to establish new neural networks for joy and well-being.

Using this program, you can develop the gifts once ascribed only to a privileged few. And in the process, you'll have the chance to gain other health benefits, including a reduced risk of devastating brain diseases, cancer, heart disease, and Parkinson's; elimination of debilitating mood swings; the breaking of unhealthy emotional and behavior patterns; the overcoming of painful memories and past traumas; a powerful clarity of thought; and the potential for maximum human life span; all without the use of drugs.

When we repair our brains and heal our toxic emotions, we move toward a state of personal health and well-being. Then, we can bring forth the qualities attributed to enlightened beings: inner peace, wisdom, compassion, joy, creativity, and a new vision of the future.

CHAPTER 1

THE NEUROSCIENCE OF ENLIGHTENMENT

Can neuroscience deliver on the promises presented by religion: freedom from suffering, violence, scarcity, and disease? Can neuroscience deliver us into a life where health, peace, and abundance reign?

The pledges of the world's religions are so universal that it's likely the longing for joy, inner peace, and well-being are hardwired into the human brain and have become a social instinct as powerful as the drive to procreate. The Bible, the Koran, and Buddhist and Hindu scriptures all teach that we can be delivered into a paradisiacal state, whether after death, at the end of time, following many reincarnations, or as a result of personal effort and merit. This state of liberation is called grace or Heaven by Christian religions, Paradise by Muslims, while Eastern traditions refer to it as awakening or enlightenment, using various terms such as *samadhi, mukti, bodhi, satori,* and *nirvana.*

But what if grace, samadhi, and enlightenment are really based in biological science? What if they are states of higher order and complexity created by programmable circuits in the brain? What if these circuits could make it possible to attain lifelong joy, inner

1

peace, health, and well-being now, in this physical world, and not in some distant future or afterlife?

THE ENERGY MATRIX

In the 1930s, Dogon shamans of western Africa informed two French anthropologists of the existence of a companion sun to Sirius, the Dog Star. This celestial body could not be seen with the naked eye, and the shamans had no access to sophisticated telescopes. Yet they described it as extremely heavy, orbiting around Sirius in an elliptical pattern that required half a century for each complete cycle. Forty years later, astronomers with powerful telescopes identified the star and named it Sirius B.[1]

There are many more examples of the discovery of seemingly impossible knowledge. For example, Amazon sages claimed that, after fasting and praying during vision quests, they were taught by the plants themselves how to prepare curare, a neurotoxin employed for hunting and also used for modern anesthesia.

Curare contains deadly poisons from the bark of *Strychnos toxifera* and from moonseed flowers, in particular from *Chondrodendron tomentosum*. The most common method of preparation is to slowly cook the bark scrapings of *Strychnos* and moonseed for exactly 75 hours, after which the mixture becomes a dark, syrupy paste. During cooking, if its sweet-scented vapors were to be inhaled, the muscles involved in respiration would relax and cease to respond, resulting in instant death from asphyxiation. The men who prepare it watch it cook from a safe distance so as to avoid inhaling its fumes. A victim of curare poisoning is horribly aware of not breathing and lucidly witnesses the body going into convulsions while being unable to move or call for help. Amazingly, however, *after* curare is cooked, it can be safely touched and rolled into a paste that is harmless even if swallowed. But if curare comes into direct contact with the bloodstream, it is deadly—as when the poison is applied to arrow tips that pierce the skin of victims. How could the shamans have known about this effect? It is statistically impossible to discover the formula for curare through trial and error, which underlines the shamans' claim that they accessed information from the natural world—from the biosphere itself—by tapping into the invisible wisdom of a field that permeates all of life. This web of life, which they refer to as the Divine Mother, is a living energy system that supports and informs all creatures. It is, in essence, a matrix of energy that connects all living entities. This concept is making its way back into the minds of the science community. Scientists are also beginning to reconsider the notion of space as one huge void. Instead, a growing number of physicists postulate that space is not empty but full of energy: cosmic radiation from the Big Bang, pulsating electromagnetic fields, and gravity. Could this energy be a vast storehouse of information as well?

THE FEMININE THROUGH HISTORY

Ancient peoples recognized and revered the power of the divine feminine in her many forms, such as the Divine Mother of the shamans. For millennia, before the advent of the alphabet, cultures around the world, from the Indus Valley to Central Europe, celebrated the Goddess. In India, Kali has long been worshipped as the Great Mother and the ultimate reality. In Greece, Hera represented a much older mother deity, perhaps related to the Sumerian goddess Inanna, while the goddess Demeter, revered in the Eleusinian Mysteries, was the Great Mother of planting and harvesting crops.

Throughout Central Europe, the earliest of representations of the Great Mother are stone and bone pieces collectively referred to as Venus figurines. The best known of these is the Venus of Willendorf, a symbol of fertility with large breasts and hips, named after the village in central Austria near which it was found. This statuette was carved close to 25,000 years ago from limestone and tinted with red ocher that is not native to the area, suggesting that it had perhaps been a treasured possession brought from elsewhere by a pilgrim. Similar figurines have been found throughout the area and in such great numbers that some anthropologists are convinced they point to a time when the feminine form was the singular representation of the Divine.

Marija Gimbutas, an archeologist known for her research into the Neolithic cultures of Europe, offers compelling evidence that the European heartland was once invaded by Indo-European peoples from what is today the Ukraine and southern Russia. Being fierce warriors, these invaders rode newly domesticated horses and easily defeated the Goddess-worshipping Neolithic farmers. These invaders were known as members of the Battle Ax culture because they characteristically placed a stone battle ax, which by that time was useless as a weapon but held only symbolic value, in the graves of males.

When the Battle Ax people arrived in Europe around 3000 B.C.E., they replaced the mythologies of the Great Mother with those of a male deity, and the representation of the Divine became the phallus or the tree of life. The chief deity in the Indo-European pantheon is Dyeus, God of the Sky, who was addressed as Father Sky or Shining Father. The name Dyeus is the root of the Latin word for deity, *deus*. In Greece, Dyeus would become Zeus and, in Rome, Jupiter.

THE LOSS OF THE FEMININE

With the first Sumerian cuneiform tablets, Indus script, and Egyptian hieroglyphs around 3000–2500 B.C.E., at the start of the Bronze Age, scribes of that period began to record the stories of military leaders and the songs of poets. Accounts of historical events became regarded as undisputed fact and began to replace legends, which were a mixture of fact and myth conveyed from one generation to the next through a rich oral tradition. Male gods of the sky and heavens, such as Zeus, Yahweh, Thor, and Shiva, took dominance over goddess traditions and the earth goddesses.

People no longer saw nature as the manifestation of divinity but as a resource: forests were for building houses and ships, soil was to be tilled for crops, and animals were to be bred for food. A mechanistic view of nature began to prevail as alchemists gave way to chemists and astrologers to astronomers. With the arrival of Newtonian physics in the late 1600s, any force that couldn't be explained by science was dismissed as superstition.

Western medicine was born of this worldview. Instead of relying on natural remedies to cure the ailments of the body, physicians turned to synthetic drugs and surgery. The scientific worldview replaced the mysterious world of the ancients. The invention of microscopes enabled scientists to investigate what were once deemed invisible "spirits" that cause disease and to catalogue them as microbes.

Later, investigators discovered the genetic code and began to entertain the notion that mortal humans could control health in the same way they controlled nature. Geneticists and chemists found ways to manipulate genes and conquer disease with prescription drugs.

These days, Western physicians seem overly focused on reflexively responding to physical problems that they believe underlie their patients' maladies. Whether the cause is a smoldering infectious agent or a chemical imbalance, all too often both physician and patient regard the prescription pad as the sole means to treat a disease, thus ignoring the more fundamental issue of patient uniqueness.

A RETURN TO THE FEMININE

And yet, the pendulum has begun to swing back to the belief in an interconnected universe and the importance of the divine feminine. Contemporary scientists, including the Noble Prize–winner Erwin Schrödinger, the neuroscientist Humberto Maturana, and the physicist Francisco Varela, have suggested the interrelatedness of all particles in the universe.

We can find evidence of this interconnectedness in physics in a property known as entanglement. Evidence indicates that when two particles are created together, such as through the radioactive decay of other particles, they remain linked together, or entangled, no matter how far apart they might be from each other.

Variables in the condition of each particle remain undetermined until they are observed and measured. For example, when one entangled particle has a positive charge, its mate will have a negative charge. Reversing the charge of one causes an instantaneous reversal in the other. This defies the laws of General Relativity because it would involve a signal traveling faster than the speed of light. Yet the concept of entanglement is consistent with the laws of quantum mechanics, which describe a universe in which distant interactions are not only permitted but commonplace. Quantum mechanics is thought to apply only to subatomic particles because quantum effects are not observable on a larger scale. But Stuart Hameroff, an anesthesiologist and professor at the University of Arizona, and Jack A. Tuszynski, a physicist at the University of Alberta, both suggest that quantum processing—on a level larger than subatomic—may actually be occurring inside the brain.[2]

A commonly accepted scientific model states that consciousness arises as the result of the computational power—the information processing capabilities—of the human brain. Hameroff is studying microtubules, which are structural components of the cell that transport nutrients from the cell body to the axon terminal. In Hameroff's research, he noted that anesthesia works through an effect on neural microtubules. The correlation between consciousness and computational power led Hameroff to reason that these microtubules could, in fact, act as information-processing modules, which would increase the current estimates of human computational capabilities more than a millionfold. And if this were the case, simple computing power could offer humans the mental "bandwidth" necessary to commune consciously with the biosphere—in essence tapping into the information of our interconnected universe. With research such as this, scientists are finding models to elucidate what shamans and seers have so elegantly and simply explained in the past as our ability to have an active dialogue with all of nature.

YOUR COMPUTATIONAL MIND

The number of neurons in the brain is 10 to the 11th power—that's a 1 followed by 11 zeroes, or 100 billion! With close to 10,000 synapses in every large neuron and with switch rates close to 1,000 times per second, this means that the number of operations the brain can process per second is 10 to the 18th power.[3] While this is an incredibly large number, it becomes minute if neuronal microtubules are involved as computational subunits. With more than 100 million microtubules in each neuron, the increased computational capability of the brain becomes staggeringly immense.

But whether the number of computations the human brain can perform is a 10 followed by 18 zeroes or a 10 followed by 27 zeroes is not as consequential as how well we are using the brain we have now. If we were to ask you to remember the song "Hey Jude" for a moment and then ask you to forget it, you, in common with most people, would have a hard time putting it out of your mind. Regardless of the possible number of computations our brain is capable of, the truth of the matter is that most people use most of their computational ability to dwell on everyday problems. This waste of a good brain leaves hardly any computational power for innovation, creative problem solving, and enlightenment.

If Hameroff is right about microtubules exhibiting quantum mechanical events inside your brain cells, then consider the possibilities and potentials that you are capable of, especially when you turn off thoughts of fear, sex, greed, or incessant worry. You could have the power to engage in nonlocal interactions, to access information from across the galaxy, and to draw upon the lessons from your past, your future, or even from the collective past and future of humanity—just as enlightened meditators and shamans do and have done. As the Dalai Lama states, "Those on a high level of spiritual experience have . . . developed meditative concentration to the point of becoming clairvoyant and generating miracles."[4]

THE BRAIN AND ENLIGHTENMENT

So with all this expanded brain power, what are we striving for? In the East, enlightenment has traditionally been associated with qualities such as generosity, compassion, peaceful acceptance, and an experience of oneness with all creation. In the fiercely individualistic West, our rather vague notion of enlightenment suggests an acceptance of the world as it is, or of discovering how we can change it for the better. Enlightenment for us also implies the common longing for novelty, exploration, and creativity, as personified by the explorers who venture into space.

If we take the Eastern qualities of enlightenment out of their religious context and place them in the realm of biological science, we find that they are attributes associated with the activation of the prefrontal cortex—the newest part of the human brain. On functional MRI scans, people who meditate regularly are shown to have developed brains that are *wired* differently than the brains of people who don't meditate. They are better able to remain calm and stress-free, live in peace, and practice compassion. Curiously, their prefrontal cortex is the most active region in their brain during the states they describe as samadhi, or enlightenment. His Holiness the Dalai Lama describes enlightenment as "a state of freedom not only from the counterproductive emotions that drive the process of cyclic existence, but also from the predispositions established in the mind by those afflictive emotions."[5] The Dalai Lama is suggesting that enlightenment is a state of freedom from destructive emotions and from the limiting beliefs and repetitive behaviors created by these emotions.

Generosity and compassion arise only when the prefrontal cortex is able to throttle back the more prehistoric regions of the brain. Yet, for the prefrontal cortex to create functional pathways for joy and peace, the entire body and brain need to be healthy, fed with the proper nutrients, and trained with an inner discipline. We must heal our bodies and minds to empower the prefrontal cortex—the new brain, which is biologically programmable for bliss, extraordinary longevity, peace, and regeneration. For too long, this brain region has been kept offline, silenced by the same forces—scarcity, violence, and trauma—from which it promises to deliver us.

Once this new region in the brain is brought online, brain synergy is possible. Synergy means that the whole is greater than the sum of its parts. Engineers are familiar with how synergy operates. The tensile strength of stainless steel, for example, is nearly ten times greater than the tensile strength of iron, even though stainless steel is basically iron with a minute amount of carbon added to it. Both carbon and iron, by themselves, are brittle and flake easily. Yet, when combined, they make an extraordinarily strong material.

Brain synergy signifies a neurocomputer whose circuits are all turned on, tuned in, and operating collaboratively, each region attending to its functions—much as the heart attends to circulating blood while the lungs attend to respiration—creating a system that cannot be defined or even described by its component parts.

ATTAINING SYNERGY

People in the East say the path to brain synergy is through the practice of meditation. Shamans use the term *clear perception*. In yoga, it is called samadhi, the highest stage of meditation, oneness with the universe. Regardless of the term used to describe the process, the challenge is to *dis-identify with your limited sense of self that was created by destructive emotions*.

Think of a lake. When the waters of the lake are still, it reflects everything around it perfectly. You see pine trees on the other side or a rising moon as mirror images. But when even the slightest breeze crosses the lake, the surface reflects only itself. It, in effect, says, "Look at me." Similarly, when your mind is disrupted by uninvited thoughts or emotions or when it is distracted by television or a barrage of commercial advertising or social gossip or trivial banter, it removes itself from connection with the greater universe. It interrupts your deep, innate desire to perceive the grand mystery of creation—and be part of it. Shamans believe that, to interact with the vast information fields of the biosphere, you must enter a state of clear perception. Your mind must be at peace in order to perceive the true nature of the world and not merely the reflection of your own below-the-surface drama created by your destructive emotions.

A teaching story from the North American Plains Indians tells of a young man who comes to his grandfather and says, "There are two wolves inside of me. One wants to kill and destroy, and the other one wants to make peace and bring beauty. Which one will win, Grandfather?" The old man answers, "Whichever one you feed."

Likewise, you have a choice: To feed the wolf of chaos and confusion, the wolf that devours your positive thinking, destroys your sense of self-worth, and consumes your entire being. Or to feed the wolf of inner peace that will enable your mind to become like the beautiful, reflective surface of a still lake and access the attributes and gifts of your higher brain.

Once you heal your emotional brain and create the state of brain synergy, the gifts of your prefrontal cortex will come online naturally. You will no longer need to pursue happiness through artificial means, because *happiness will arise from you* with ease. For the prefrontal cortex, happiness is not the result of good luck or happenstance. No, happiness is a treasure of clear perception that will be eternally yours.

CHAPTER 2

THE POWERFUL MIND

In our work—both as an anthropologist who dedicated many years to investigating the healing practices of Amazon and Andean sages, and as a neurologist who has spent decades treating individuals suffering from degenerative brain diseases—we have long been intrigued by the power of the mind in achieving unbelievable feats, both physical and mental. We've met and studied with sages who were able to achieve extraordinary brilliance, inner peace, and creativity. We've heard of Tibetan monks who are able to meditate overnight on an ice-covered mountain without freezing to death, dusting the snow from their naked shoulders as the sun rises.

The full power of the mind is still not completely understood, but we witness examples of it on a regular basis.

HEALTH AND THOUGHTS

Years ago, people saw support groups and stress management techniques as harmless adjuncts to the medical treatment of those with serious illnesses. Recently, however, research has shown that patients who use techniques such as mindful meditation not only are less stressed emotionally by their illness but also experience better physical health. This research is, in fact, showing how thoughts, beliefs, and emotions influence the health of the body.

In the July 2009 issue of *Scientific American*, the neurologist Martin Portner describes the case of Gretchen, a participant in a 2005 study on the viability of a testosterone patch to treat hypoactive sexual desire disorder, a condition in which a person's libido is so diminished that he or she feels no sexual interest or attraction. Testosterone, a hormone produced by the testes in males and the ovaries in females, is associated with sexual arousal. Gretchen had felt no sexual desire ever since undergoing an operation that removed her ovaries.

After wearing the patch for 12 weeks, Gretchen felt the stirrings of desire again. "It can only be because of that patch," she reported. Shortly thereafter she was able to make love with her husband again and experience an orgasm for the first time in years. But the most amazing part of the story is that Gretchen, unbeknownst to her, was part of the study's control group and the patch given to her was a placebo with no testosterone in it whatsoever.

The return of Gretchen's sexual appetite was clearly related to a change in her neural wiring, some literal *change of mind* of which she was not even cognitively aware. Yet, it happened. And that change was felt throughout her body.

Most of us are more familiar with psychosomatic disease than with psychosomatic wellness. We know that we can worry ourselves sick, and we suspect that we can laugh ourselves to health. Even so, medicine gives little credence to the idea that psychosomatic health can be achieved. After all, we cannot knowingly administer a placebo to ourselves, in the same way that it is impossible to tickle yourself. Yet societies that rely on traditional healers—medicine men and women—have long understood the power of the mind to either heal or kill. At times, shamans resort to great pomp and ceremony to mobilize the mind's ability to heal the body. Their complex ceremonies activate the prefrontal cortex to create health.

Yet, in modern societies, we have largely declared these practices to be superstition or quackery; "placebo" is even a term of dismissal in everyday conversation. The irony is that our modern-day "ceremony" consists of giving the patient a sugar pill, a tablet that contains no pharmaceutical ingredients. Testing new medicines against a placebo is a common practice for determining the efficacy of all medications, which is, in effect, strong evidence that the mind alone does have the power to soothe inflammation, calm nerves, and influence organs and tissues of the body to return to a state of health.

Studies have shown, for example, that a sugar pill can be as effective as morphine in 56 percent of people.[1] Yet, even though the sugar pill is the most carefully studied "medication" by manufacturers and researchers of pharmaceutical medicine, it is the one least appreciated or recognized as a potential cure.

A friend of ours once suggested that if we wanted to get rich we should press chicken soup into pill form and sell it over the counter with the name "Placebo," as we could make legitimate scientific claims that it would be almost as effective as expensive medications in treating a host of complaints, ranging from headaches to erectile dysfunction.

The placebo effect and psychosomatic wellness are the result of tapping into the healing potential of the mind, which has been common practice in humankind for thousands of years. By dismissing the placebo effect, Western medicine has, in reality, failed to investigate how this phenomenon can give us a glimpse into the immense power of the prefrontal cortex.

■ ■ ■

David:
Cancer? What Cancer?

As a trained neurologist, I'm intrigued by how I am often accused of practicing "nontraditional" medicine because, in addition to offering nutritional recommendations, our clinic's protocols also incorporate such modalities as affirmations and meditation. The paradox is that these practices, or similar ones, have been a part of health care for thousands of years, and are thus "traditional" by definition.

In late 2007, a patient with a very serious health issue came to see me. "Marvin" was a 74-year-old man who had just returned from a top cancer treatment facility, where he was told to "get your affairs in order" because he had been diagnosed with aggressive pancreatic cancer that had already spread to the adjacent lymph nodes. Chemotherapy was an option, but the success rate, especially at his age, was almost zero percent. Given what modern medicine has to offer someone in Marvin's condition, the cancer specialists had told him what they assessed to be the truth about his devastating illness: he had, at best, about six months to live.

Knowing how much of an impact beliefs have on physical health, I asked him if he truly believed that, and he replied, "Absolutely not!"—which was exactly the response I was hoping for.

Working with my team, we therefore designed a program of specific nutritional supplements to enhance his immune system. I also added a high-dosage DHA to augment the meditation practices and affirmations he was to begin. The focus of both of these techniques was simply the thought, "I am healthy."

Within one week, his previous sallow appearance had disappeared, and remarkably, within six weeks, his previously abnormal blood studies related to pancreatic and liver function had completely normalized. Three months later, he returned to the renowned hospital where he'd been diagnosed. His CAT scans revealed no evidence of cancer whatsoever.

"What did they say when they saw your results?" I asked him.

"Well," he replied, "they really didn't seem interested in learning what I was doing, but they did say that whatever it was, I should continue it."

Almost two years later, at the time of writing this book, Marvin remains cancer-free. Sure, it could be argued that this is simply a case of spontaneous remission, but that is exceedingly rare with this type of cancer, as any cancer specialist would confirm. I submit that the key intervention was the relationship he cultivated with the Divine as a result of using the two-pronged approach of neuronutrients and shamanic meditative techniques that allowed him to access the healing energy that infuses all that exists.

■ ■ ■

In contrast to the placebo, the nocebo is an insidious complement. A nocebo is an otherwise harmless substance or inert medication that can cause harmful effects due to the patient's negative expectations, beliefs, or psychological condition—regardless of the person's physical condition.

■ ■ ■

Alberto:
The Curse Is Real

The most dramatic example of the nocebo effect I ever witnessed occurred in the Peruvian Amazon when I met a perfectly healthy man who had been "cursed" by a local sorcerer. At the time, I was investigating the healing practices of shamans near the headwaters of the Marañón River. When the patient came in for a consultation, the healer informed the patient that his nausea and headaches were being caused by this curse, that there was nothing he could do to help him, and that he should prepare himself and his family for his passing. Within 24 hours the man was dead. When I asked the healer why he had not helped the man, he replied that the man had broken a village taboo but it was his own fear that had killed him. I immediately questioned him further, asking if the curse was all in the man's own mind, that the sorcery was not real. "Oh no," he emphasized. "The curse, the sorcery, is absolutely real."

What I learned in that corner of the Amazon was the same thing that advertising agencies on Madison Avenue have long understood: that the mind can be programmed to purchase vehicles that will make us feel like we are young again and dresses that promise to make the hurt of depression go away. The mind can even be programmed to go against every instinctual survival function ingrained through millions of years of evolution. It is very difficult to override the body's immune system. Yet that man's belief had managed to kill him. The question that came to my mind that day was: What about the long list of disclaimers and possible side effects that come with every medication we buy? Could they be affecting our very suggestible minds in a noxious way? Rather than falling prey to nocebos—whether of the physical body or mind—how can we program ourselves for life, health, and joy?

I have since come to realize that physicians are hesitant to suggest a placebo or to recommend what were once called "soft therapies," such as counseling, relaxation techniques, or meditation, because they believe these methodologies constitute phony medicine. They worry about the implications of "tricking" the patient into healing the body, even though the success of many medically accepted therapies and surgical interventions currently performed by those same doctors may be, in large part, enhanced or facilitated by the placebo effect.

But above all, as I have come to understand the capabilities of our mind, I realize that you and I and everyone can use these faculties consciously to create psychosomatic health. In effect, we will be able to volitionally heal ourselves from physical and emotional disorders, without having to resort to trickery. To do this, we first have to understand how the brain works, and how trauma can injure the brain regions that allow us to tap into these abilities.

■ ■ ■

THE TRIUNE BRAIN

In the mid-1950s, Paul D. MacLean, an American neuroscientist, proposed a model to help explain the evolution of the human brain. MacLean's model became known as the triune brain, and it describes how we have three evolutionarily distinct neurocomputers, each with its own intelligence, subjective feel of the world, and sense of time and space. MacLean's model is too general to be of value to students of evolutionary anatomy, yet it is helpful to metaphorically understand how each of us reacts differently to situations, depending on the "brain" we are responding from. It explains how, when we smell the scent of wolf, one of us may sense danger while the other may detect opportunity.

The Old Brains

The first brain is the reptilian brain, or R-brain, which is anatomically very similar to the brain of modern-day reptiles. This brain region is completely instinctual and is primarily interested in survival. It regulates most autonomic functions, such as breathing, heart rate, and body temperature; and it is involved in the fight-or-flight response. There is nothing cuddly about a reptile, and this brain region, like a cold-blooded serpent, feels no emotions.

The second brain is the limbic system, which is made up primarily of the amygdala, the hypothalamus, and the hippocampus. MacLean described this as the brain of instinct and emotion. The limbic system is also known as the mammalian brain, or M-brain. As the name implies, this is the brain most dominant in mammals, which flourished about the same time that dinosaurs were staving off extinction. As such, it represents one more step in the ladder of evolutionary complexity.

In the limbic system, signals are decoded according to four fundamental programs, known as the Four F's—fear, feeding, fighting, and fornicating. The M-brain will interpret meeting a person for the first time as an individual to be wary of, a dinner date or a promising business partner, a potential adversary, or a possible mate. This brain also interprets color according to the cultural environment that programmed it: red, for example, means "danger, stop" in the United States, but it means "good fortune" to the people of China, and "best" or "beautiful" to Russians.

Anatomy of the Limbic Brain

To better understand how the limbic, or mammalian, brain functions, let's look at the structures within it that evolved to ensure our survival. The limbic brain contains the seahorse-shaped hippocampus and the almond-shaped amygdala. Both are involved in processing information from our environment via our emotions. If an enemy ambushes us, we become terrified and fight or flee. If a snake strikes out at us, we instinctively jump away.

The hippocampus is located in the deepest and most forward portion of each medial temporal lobe and extends into both hemispheres of the brain. The hippocampus received its name in the 16th century when Italian anatomist Julius Caesar Aranzi noted its uncanny resemblance to the seahorse and chose the name *hippocampus,* the Greek word for this creature.

Early researchers, attempting to ascribe particular functions to specific brain areas, believed the hippocampus was involved with olfaction, the perception of smell. No doubt this belief was strengthened by the location of the hippocampus near the olfactory system. Even though research later showed that olfaction was not a primary function of the hippocampus, investigators continue to explore the relationship between the memory of scents and hippocampal function. Notice how a familiar smell will remind you of your childhood, such as a whiff of sizzling bacon that evokes the breakfasts your mother used to make.

More refined research today, however, reveals that, rather than serving as a storage center for memories, the hippocampus acts more as a way station, acquiring information from the five senses and then parceling out the data for processing either by the amygdala, in the event of a perceived threat, or to the cerebral cortex for all other needs.

In effect, the hippocampus operates something like a digital camera that can process both still pictures and video. Facts, like photographs, are pieces of data that can generally be verbalized in simple terms. Recalling facts is termed declarative memory. Events, like video, are more complex and involve relationships that are both spatial as well as temporal. This mental activity is called episodic memory.

When the hippocampus begins to deteriorate, new experiences are less likely to be stored and memorialized, and this is a hallmark of Alzheimer's disease. Advanced imaging techniques like MRI and PET scans now clearly show that loss of physical tissue as well as loss of function in the hippocampus is an early indicator of this disease.

As you'll see later in *Power Up Your Brain*, the hippocampus begins to fail due to free radical and chemical damage caused by trauma and stress. Basically, once the hippocampus begins to fail, school is over and learning pretty much stops. Conventional wisdom believes that the ability to process information through higher brain centers is stunted, that our emotional repertoire is diminished, and that genuine feelings become inaccessible.

Our mission, however, is to challenge that paradigm and demonstrate to you that neurodegeneration is preventable and even reversible. Ring the bell. School is back in session.

The amygdala, from the Greek word for *almond,* governs our so-called fight-or-flight response, which is our automatic and instantaneous reaction to real or imagined threats. Basically, it's the fear center of the brain that allows us to respond to dangerous situations reflexively, unconsciously, and immediately.

The New Brain

The third brain identified by MacLean is the neocortex, which is well developed in all the higher mammals and is responsible for speech, writing, and higher-order thinking in humans. If we do not need to fear, fight, seduce, or dine with a person we encounter in any particular situation, the thalamus relays the sensory information, colored by the joys, excitements, worries, or concerns of the limbic brain, to the neocortex for reflection and appropriate behavior.

The neocortex processes signals in a holistic fashion, interpreting environmental sights and sounds into coherent messages. Through the neocortex, we recognize the value of all people and set aside any thoughts about how they could be useful to us or what we might be able to get from them, either legally or illegally. The neocortex reminds us to call friends for no reason other than to say hello and wish them well and not only when we need to ask a favor.

It is in these higher cortical areas that selfless love, reasoning, and logic take place. This brain allows us to create new ideas and entertain notions such as democracy as well as to understand mathematics, write poetry, compose music and art, dream of freedom, and envision the future.

Our two older neurocomputers, the R-brain and the limbic system, think primarily in terms of distance to the kill, how far back to the village of origin, the friendly confines of the childhood home, and personal space. They recognize spatial boundaries associated with relationships, the blood family, clan territory, ethnic neighborhoods, and national borders. With these anchors firmly embedded in memory, the primordial brains can easily identify what is "my area" and what is "their land." These brains believe that good fences make good neighbors and perceive "those people over there" to be "others" and "not our kind." They associate people with places, which is helpful knowledge to ensure survival but limiting to the concept of a global community. Consider how easily you can forget someone's name but remember the face. That situation stems from your primitive brain's ability to draw upon memory and emotion in order to discern between "the bad guys on the other side of the tracks" and "the good guys who are like us."

In contrast, the neocortex, associated with the higher executive functions, is able to think in terms of time and not only of space. It can store food for the winter, plan an irrigation canal for the dry season, and anticipate where the herd might go for the spring. It will mark the turning of seasons and have an inclination for mathematics and music. This brain is able to plan and recognize future actions and consequences, to choose between good and bad, right and wrong, and to suppress socially incorrect behaviors and responses. The neocortex can restrain the Four F's of the limbic brain and is involved in meditative and transcendental experiences.

Perhaps it is the neocortex's ability to comprehend our limited time on earth that generates a fear of death and keeps many of us from exploring its potentials. The limbic brain understands that death happens in the same primal way that children know that kittens and grandparents die. But the limbic brain does not realize that death will happen to *us* and somehow imagines that we are immune from it. This, coupled with the fact that the developing brain is more prone to risk-taking behavior, is why some teenagers act as though the laws of gravity and centrifugal force do not apply to them as they speed with a carload of friends along a winding mountain road after drinking too much

If you have not awakened your neocortical gifts in your youth, they will tend to remain dormant until much later in life, only to awaken reluctantly. By the age of 40, most of us have grown to accept that we may not have a second chance at youth. Perhaps this is why, for instance, Orthodox rabbis traditionally warned against the study of mystical texts until age 40, when maturity was more likely to be accompanied by wisdom. Likewise, life insurance salespeople know it is nearly impossible to sell a policy to anyone who does not yet recognize that their time will run out and that every moment is precious; until that stage of practical enlightenment, which happens around age 40, these persons are convinced that death will not happen to them.

Advanced Neocortical Thinking

Synesthesia, which is the ability to blend senses, is one of the many faculties of the neocortex. Artists and musicians possess this quality, which enables them to see a V of flying geese at a distance, imagine the sound of their flapping wings, then set that aural and visual composition to music or canvas. Even in common language, we sometimes use synesthetic or cross-sensory descriptors to create juxtapositional idioms, such as a "bitter wind" or a "loud color."

Daniel Tammet, an English savant, is one person who expresses synesthetic capability literally to the nth degree. Tammet can, for example, recite the mathematical constant pi from memory to 22,514 decimal places and divide 97 by 13 with complete accuracy to over 100 decimal places. In his best-selling book

Born on a Blue Day: Inside the Extraordinary Mind of an Autistic Savant, Tammet describes how he thinks.

He says that when he performs a mathematical calculation, such as multiplying 37 to the power of 4, which he can do faster than you can press the numbers on a calculator, the answer comes to him in a rich, kaleidoscopic confluence of colors, textures, shapes, hues, and feelings.

Tammet was diagnosed as having high-functioning autism. He developed his extraordinary capabilities after a series of epileptic seizures during childhood that may have rewired his brain, allowing him to tap into a limited range—a deep but narrow slice—of his neocortical capabilities. Daniel's experience is not unlike that of sages in the high Andes who claim that extraordinary telepathic and clairvoyant skills appeared shortly after they were struck by lightning or after a strenuous vision quest of fasting and praying for numerous days.

Daniel Tammet's gifts are not limited to mathematics. He also has the ability to learn a new language within a short period of time. For a television special, he mastered the complex and difficult Icelandic language—which contains, for example, 12 words for each of the numbers one, two, three, and four, depending on the context, and a strict adherence to gender agreement between nouns and adjectives—in less than a week. This enabled him to conduct a live interview on Icelandic television in the native language, a task that he performed flawlessly.

Some investigators argue that such great gifts come at a great price; they say that nearly 50 percent of all savants are also autistic. This has led Wisconsin psychiatrist and investigator Darold Treffert to suggest that savant syndrome is caused by damage to the left brain hemisphere, particularly the frontal areas, which causes the right hemisphere to overcompensate.[2]

This is said by Dr. Treffert to be accompanied by a shift from high-level frontal lobe memory and processing to low-level procedural memory, which allows persons like Daniel Tammet to master numbers and languages with such ease.

CHAPTER 3

THE EVOLUTION OF THE BRAIN AND THE MIND

Thousands of years ago, our ancestors faced a neurological opportunity similar to the one we face today, an opportunity that facilitated an evolutionary leap forward. With the awakening of the neocortex, our forebears acquired a new brain structure that nature had wired for joy, creativity, and innovation.

To access that potential, our ancestors required specific nutrients to provide fuel to run their neurocomputer. Once they added brain-enriching foods to their diet, the faculties of certain individuals, the visionaries of their day, came online and began to create great works of art, devise written language, establish civilizations, and lay the foundations for our modern human experience.

During this time, ancestral shamans described Creation as a web of life in which we are all interconnected. This was a kind of Indra's Net, which the mythology of ancient India describes as a web with an infinite number of intersecting strands and a precious jewel at the intersection of every strand. Each of the infinite number of jewels reflects every other jewel perfectly. Within this mythical net, all beings are interrelated, and all of our actions, no matter how slight, affect everyone else. Within this net, prophets converse with God and interpret His will, while mystics search for the elixir of immortality and alchemists attempt to transform lead into gold. These sages, mystics, and alchemists shared the same preoccupations as seers of today. They asked, as we do now: How can we live long and healthy lives, unaffected by debilitating illness and degenerative brain disease? How can we turn the dense *lead of human suffering* into the *gold of enlightened consciousness*?

In the scheme of history, the quest for metaphysical answers about the origin of life died when Charles Darwin published *The Origin of Species.* The popular understanding of the time was that life is a perennial struggle for survival, that humankind is governed by a harsh Law of the Jungle where only the fittest win.

But, fortunately, after centuries of scientists' dismissal and ignoring of the ancient teachings, people in all walks of life are once again asking the mystic's questions about the significance and potential of human consciousness. Could evolution have also been favoring the survival of the wisest?

WAYS OF FEAR, WAYS OF WISDOM

The history of human consciousness is marked by the battle between the older awareness, *the ways of fear*, and the newer awareness, *the ways of love.* When the newer awareness prevails, we discover a God of love and compassion, express religious freedom, and practice generosity. When the older awareness dominates, we tend to worship an angry god who scourges his enemies with plagues and who sends his chosen people on so-called holy wars to ensure his dominance. With the older brain, greed and intolerance prevail.

Lower awareness views everything, even nature's beauty and bounty, as a commodity, valued only as a means to generate profit. Water, one of the essential elements of life, is seen not as a home of aquatic organisms and a natural means of transportation but as a liquid to be bottled and sold. Air, another essential element, is seen not as a vital substance indispensable for breath but as vacant space in which to emit industrial waste products. Soil is seen not as a necessity for growing food but as property to be owned, fenced, and contaminated with agricultural chemicals and industrial and domestic waste. Mountains are seen not for their majesty but as places to be stripped of minerals and ores. Forests are seen not as animal habitats and places for spiritual retreat but as potential planks and boards. Even space beyond the sky above is seen not just as an opportunity for galactic exploration but as a place to dump planetary trash and spy on our global neighbors.

Even human beings are viewed as a commodity when our thinking is fettered to the ways of fear. Children in developing nations, for example, are seen as labor pawns in sweatshops or, in developed countries, as future rank-and-file employees. Senior citizens, at least in Western societies, are not revered for their wisdom but warehoused in "old people's homes" until death finally gets them out of the way. People of ages in between, according to Darwinian protocol, are often trained in warfare or programmed to "get even," if not "get ahead," even at the expense of other fellow humans. But perhaps the worst dismissal of human value occurs in the spinmeister term "collateral damage," which would have us heartlessly gloss over the killing of innocent civilians who happen to be caught in a war zone.

And while the new, higher awareness offers us the ability to think on a sophisticated and grand scale—to see Earth from space and to comprehend that, as the health of the planet goes, so goes our own health and well-being—we find societies, whether developed or emerging, returning again and again to seemingly inevitable violence in order to resolve conflicts and impose values on others.

While arguments wage over global warming—whether it exists or not and, if so, who is to blame, and what is the cause and the cure—and whether or not the world is perched on the edge of ecological disaster, many individuals are beginning to realize that human society is also standing on the brink of an extraordinary leap in consciousness.

In the previous chapter, we carefully looked at the characteristics of the brain's first three evolutionary stages: that is, the reptilian or R-brain, the limbic system, and the neocortex. Now, to understand this extraordinary leap and to better manifest the opportunity at hand, we need to look more closely at the development of the fourth brain—the prefrontal cortex.

THE PREFRONTAL CORTEX: KEY TO ENLIGHTENMENT

In humans, the prefrontal cortex, located in the front of the brain, takes on critically important significance as our link to the future, our key to enlightenment, the answer to those ancient questions: How can we live long and healthy lives, unaffected by debilitating illness and degenerative brain disease? How can we turn the dense lead of human awareness into the gold of enlightened consciousness? How can we program the brain for life, health, and joy? *How will we evolve?*

The prefrontal cortex is associated with the loftier brain functions such as reasoning, inventing the alphabet and music, discovering science, and engaging in creative thinking. Many of the functions of the prefrontal cortex remain a mystery, but we know that it is associated with personal initiative and the ability to project future scenarios, and it is quite likely the place where our individuality and sense of self developed.

When our brain functions synergistically, our prefrontal cortex is fully awakened and we have the ability to develop the very highest form of intelligence and creativity *and* remain grounded and effective in the world. We understand who we are in relationship to our village and our history. Able to think originally, we recognize what holds us back from achieving a higher level of consciousness and what will help us to attain it. We recognize how we can survive *and* thrive.

Which Brain Are You Using?

Is your life a struggle for survival? Are you forever trying to make ends meet financially? Are you living hand to mouth? If so, then your reptilian brain is in the driver's seat of your cognitive apparatus.

Do you learn your lessons through difficult love relationships? Does your prince turn into a frog with a drinking problem after the honeymoon—just like your previous prince did? Are you always ending up with abusive bosses or business partners who never seem to appreciate your contributions? If so, then your emotional mammalian brain is predominantly in charge of your consciousness.

Does your intellect get in the way of your passion and joy? Are you forever analyzing things in your head? Do you fail to listen to your instinct and your intuition? Do you mistrust anything that is not proven scientifically? Are you disconnected from your feelings and insensitive to the feelings of others, even when you try not to be? If so, then you are strapped and bound to the fiendishly logical aspect of the neocortex.

Or are you flighty and ungrounded, with your head up in the clouds? Do you walk into a room and forget what you went there to do? Are you more conversant about quantum physics, the bloodline of Mary Magdalene, and international conspiracy theories than about your children's homework or what is happening in your neighborhood? If so, then your consciousness is probably in the grip of the prefrontal cortex.

If you are experiencing a predominance of any one of these brains, it is a sign that the parts of your brain are not acting in concert with each other, that those in the background at the moment are allowing another part to dominate and exhibit only its limited traits.

In actuality, to experience brain synergy, it's necessary to be aware of your financial situation and your relationships; it's good to think logically and to dream with whimsy; and it's vital to keep all of these mental activities in balance with each other.

AWAKENING THE NEW BRAIN

In the 17th century, James Ussher, Anglican Archbishop of Armagh and Primate of All Ireland, published a treatise that identified the date on which God created the world: the evening preceding Sunday, October 23, 4004 B.C.E. on the Julian calendar. Although his chronology was based on the patriarchal lineages described in Genesis and inaccurate from a scientific perspective, the Archbishop was not totally wrong. Today, while we dismiss the good Archbishop's claim as a flight of religious fancy, he did approximate the date on which the gifts of the prefrontal cortex were becoming available for large sections of humanity at the dawn of civilization and the invention of writing

But this self-awareness didn't happen overnight; rather, it took countless generations for the prefrontal cortex to become functional enough to warrant a circuitry connection with the older parts of the brain. In fact, fossil evidence of the earliest changes in this part of the brain dates back 2.5 million years ago, during the Pliocene epoch, when an early hominid called *Australopithecus africanus* lived. The enlarged cranium of *A. africanus*—a member of the "Great Apes" family, which includes humans—was more like that of modern humans than his immediate predecessors.

This means that the artists of the Altamira cave and the hunters of the Pleistocene epoch who lived 20,000 years ago had the same brain structures we have today. Yet most members of the species lacked the nutritional support and mind-body disciplines that would allow them to experience artistic creativity and scientific discovery. This is why only a few isolated individuals awakened to the potential of the prefrontal cortex. Indeed, the gifted crafted their great works of art during secretive ceremonies deep inside caves.

With the end of the last Ice Age, around 10,000 years ago, when abundant and brain-rich food supplies became available, the prefrontal cortex began to stir. During the late Neolithic period, starting around 7,000 years ago, our ancestors initiated horticulture, which ended the need to follow and harvest food from a nomadic herd. They domesticated cattle and sowed grain crops and ground the grain into cereal. They developed a curiosity for science, exploration, and perhaps even love. And they conceived of transoceanic travel; for example, Micronesian navigators built sailing canoes in which they navigated the open ocean for hundreds of miles, using only the stars for reference and arriving at islands that were not visible from their point of departure. It was around this time in history that writing and city-states emerged in many geographically disconnected societies around the globe.

At that time, as civilization emerged in the Fertile Crescent in western Asia and the sprawling city of Mohenjo-Daro rose along the Sarasvati River in what is now Pakistan, the dietary staples of the political and religious leaders came from the Himalayan rivers and the Mediterranean Sea. These were fish and mollusks rich in docosahexaenoic acid (DHA), a brain food that has become increasingly scarce in the human diet of today. DHA provided the neuronutrient boost that brought the previously installed prefrontal cortex's software online. Is it not possible that the benefits of a DHA-rich diet explain why a great Master—Jesus of Nazareth—chose simple fishermen as candidates wise enough to be his apostles, his "fishers of men"

However, while the prefrontal software was already installed in all humans of the time, the masses, though capable of tapping into the wisdom of this brain, were still struggling between two mind-sets—the old and the new.

THE OLD MIND-SET VERSUS THE NEW MIND-SET

To truly understand the conflict inside the human mind, let's compare the power of the prefrontal cortex, or new, higher brain, with the prowess of the old brain. This comparison is akin to "the ways of fear and ways of wisdom" presented earlier in this chapter. However, there we explored fear and love from the *software* perspective, that is, emotions that come from our belief systems. Here we are examining fear and love from a *hardware* perspective, that is, the physical brain that processes those emotions.

The old brain perceives the world as a frightening place, filled with rivals competing for the same scarce resources. To this brain, what matters most is survival, and it is always ready to fight or to flee. Considering that the old brain developed in mammals at a time when large, stomping dinosaurs still roamed, it is no wonder that these survival mechanisms were firmly embedded in the core of those small, fuzzy creatures that we developed from.

The old brain in humans gave rise to the belief that the spirit world is populated with fierce gods who demand sacrifice and that the physical world is prey to invisible forces that are to be appeased. In many mythologies, the earth was populated by titans, giants with extraordinary powers, who had to be defeated. The early Greeks, for example, identified 12 Titans who ruled the earth during the legendary Golden Age. In the King James Bible, God tells Moses of "a land of giants [who] dwelled therein in old time."[1] In Greek mythology, the Titans were a race of older gods whom the Olympians banished to the darkest depths of the underworld in the War of the Titans.

The old brain seeks magical and religious explanations for natural phenomena, be they the formation of mountain ranges or the course of rivers or the tempest of storms. Legends of the Inca tell of the four original beings who could move mountains and establish the course of rivers with their bare hands. Zeus, the king of the sky, wielded a thunderbolt that he periodically used to wreak havoc on the earth.

With such mythic precedent, the old brain righteously claims, "My god is stronger than your god," and believes that only those of "our faith" have been chosen for salvation, while everyone else is a pagan or a heathen destined for a hellish experience in the afterlife.

The new brain, however, understands that we do not have to live in a continuous state of threat. It knows that we are not struggling to survive in a hostile world haunted by death. It comprehends, rather, that we are all interconnected, that we can practice compassion by "turning the other cheek" and "loving our neighbors as we love ourselves," and that physical "death" is really an opportunity to return to a heavenly realm—a precept that lies at the core of the three Abrahamic religions, Judaism, Islam, and Christianity.

But even this mind-set is a matter of consciousness. At first, only those living in monastic communities and among religious orders attained this insight of the ways of wisdom. Meanwhile, the older mind-set in the majority of the populace continued to be tempted by the ways of fear. This mind-set continued to seek wealth and justify greed, while the newer, higher mind-set called out to the ways of love. These two, seemingly opposite callings have plagued humanity for millennia—and continue to do so. The disparity will only be resolved when we can turn on the truly beneficial neural programs inherent in the prefrontal cortex.

It is clear that our reasoning abilities, rooted in the more evolved brain, are not enough to prevent our suffering or give us the opportunity to create a more habitable, peaceful, and sustainable world. Indeed, if reason had ever prevailed over passion, the story of humanity would not be written in blood.

At this point in history, our species is in need of the next great opportunity offered by our prefrontal cortex, which will allow us to entertain the ancient notion of a web of life in which all creatures, and even inanimate matter, are interconnected as part of a field of information and energy. To experience enlightenment and learn to interact with this cosmic web, we must begin by healing that part of our bodies that allows us to dream a new world into being: our prefrontal cortex.

CHAPTER 4

MITOCHONDRIA AND THE FEMININE LIFE FORCE

Intricately linked to the ability of the prefrontal cortex to come fully online are the mitochondria—the powerhouses of your cells and the feminine life force referred to by shamans. Mitochondria are the conductors of the genetic orchestra that regulate how every cell ages, divides, and dies. They wave the baton that helps dictate which genes are switched on and which are switched off in every one of our cells. And they provide the fuel for establishing new neural networks. And all of the mitochondrial DNA in your body is inherited solely from your mother's lineage. That means that the source of energy that sustains your life is derived exclusively from the women in your family tree—your matrilineage.

THE POWER SOURCE WITHIN YOUR CELLS

Mitochondria were first observed by the German pathologist Richard Altmann in 1890. Seen through a microscope, these small intracellular particles look like tiny, threadlike grains. Hence the name mitochondria, derived from the Greek *mitos* meaning "thread," and *chondrin*, meaning "grain." It was not until 1949, however, that the role of mitochondria, as the producers of cellular energy, was fully explained by two biological chemistry researchers, Eugene Kennedy of the Harvard Medical School and Albert Lehninger, then of the University of Wisconsin–Madison.

Mitochondria use carbohydrates as fuel, which they convert into life-sustaining energy with the by-products of water and carbon dioxide. This process is called *oxidative metabolism*, so named because oxygen is consumed in the process, just as oxygen is consumed by fire (as demonstrated when we extinguish a flame by smothering it and depriving it of oxygen).

But, unlike in a fire, which releases energy in an uncontrolled reaction, the energy, or life force, produced by mitochondria is stored in a chemical "battery," a unique molecule called adenosine triphosphate (ATP). Energy-rich ATP can then be transported throughout the cell, releasing energy on demand in the presence of specific enzymes.[1]

In addition to the fuel they produce, mitochondria also create a by-product related to oxygen called reactive oxygen species (ROS), also known as free radicals.[2]

THE ROLE OF FREE RADICALS

These free radicals perform an important, positive function in human physiology. They play a pivotal part in regulating *apoptosis*, the process through which cells initiate self-destruction. Apoptosis happens when genetic switches that instruct a cell to die are turned on. While it may be puzzling to look upon cell death as a positive event, apoptosis is indeed a critical function that enables growth and healing of the greater organism.

Until quite recently, scientists pretty much subscribed to the paradigm that all cellular functions, including apoptosis, were directed by the cell nucleus. But, as Nick Lane notes in his compelling book, *Power, Sex, Suicide*, "there has been a change of emphasis that amounts to a revolution, overturning the nascent paradigm. The paradigm was that the nucleus is the operations centre of the cell, and controls its fate. In many respects this is of course true, but in the case of apoptosis it is not. Remarkably, cells lacking a nucleus can still commit apoptosis. The radical discovery was that the mitochondria control the fate of the cell: they determine whether a cell shall live or die."[3] Mitochondria, then, must be looked upon as being so much more than simply organelles whose job involves turning fuel into energy. They wield the Sword of Damocles.

Hippocrates was the first to use the term *apoptosis*, which literally means "the falling of leaves from a tree." However, apoptosis didn't gain traction in the scientific community until the pathologist Alastair R. Currie published an important paper describing cellular self-destruction as a basic biological phenomenon.[4] Thereafter, researchers used *apoptosis* to describe the process through which the body intentionally eliminates cells in order to serve a larger purpose.

This process begins even while the fetus is in the womb. As an example, during embryonic development, human hands initially resemble the webbed appendages of a frog. But death of the cells in the webbed area transforms these extremities, allowing for definition of individual fingers and refinement of the entire hand.

Furthermore, after birth, apoptosis is the protocol that enables your body to continuously rid itself of as many as ten billion cells every day, making room for new, healthier cells. The outcasts include a multitude of cancer cells. Most of the time, when these pathogenic cells appear, mitochondria send a signal that tells them to die rather than replicate. This is a very important mitochondrial function because runaway cancer cells don't know they need to undergo apoptosis, and, without that message from the mitochondria, they would continue to reproduce, out of control, until they endanger the host—you.

THE PROBLEM WITH FREE
RADICALS AND CELL DEATH

While cellular suicide, as described above, is generally positive, it becomes a negative situation when mitochondrial function becomes impaired and sends signals that tell normal cells to die. In fact, this is the fundamental flaw in the mitochondrial mechanism that leads to the destruction of brain cells in essentially every neurodegenerative condition, including Alzheimer's, multiple sclerosis, Parkinson's, and Lou Gehrig's disease, to name just a few. However, this brain cell apoptosis is not limited to just these diseases. The process occurs throughout your lifetime and is responsible for a general decline in brain function, even if not categorized as a disease per se.

And the catalysts—or culprits—are free radicals. Free radicals are chemicals that cause oxidative damage to tissues, essentially causing them to rust like a piece of iron left exposed to the weather. They can also damage proteins, fat, and even DNA. In fact, damage to your tissues by free radicals is thought to underlie the process of aging, a theory first described by Denham Harman, a biogerontologist who was then a research associate at the Donner Laboratory of Medical Physics at the University of California, Berkeley. His much-cited article, now considered to be a landmark work, appeared in 1956.[5]

Dr. Harman also stated that free radicals are "quenched" by antioxidants and thus laid the groundwork for an understanding of the positive effects of ingesting antioxidants, which we will learn more about later in the book.

MITOCHONDRIAL DNA

Mitochondria play a far more interesting role than simply being an energy factory and the source of ROS. Indeed, there are many characteristics of the mitochondria that serve to differentiate them from all the other structural parts of our cells. For instance, mitochondria possess their own DNA (referred to as mt-DNA), which is distinctly separate from the far more familiar and more often studied DNA in the nucleus of the cell (known as n-DNA).

While the nucleus of the cell contains exactly two copies of its DNA, mitochondria may have anywhere from two to ten copies of DNA. Interestingly, the mt-DNA, unlike n-DNA, is arranged in a ring, a configuration much like that seen in bacteria. Furthermore, in addition to similarities in the shape of their DNA, mitochondria and bacteria both lack the protein surrounding their genetic code that helps protect it from free radical damage, while in contrast, nuclear DNA is invested with protective proteins called histones, which also serve to regulate its function.

These similarities led the biologist Lynn Margulis to propose an important new theory of the origin of mitochondria.[6] She posited that mitochondria evolved hundreds of millions of years ago from aerobic (oxygen-breathing) bacteria that gradually entered into an "endosymbiotic" relationship with anaerobic bacteria, which means they began to live inside the bodies of these other organisms. This symbiosis enabled the anaerobic organisms to survive in an oxygen-rich environment. Over time, the mitochondria assumed the primary function of energy production, intracellular signaling, apoptosis regulation, and perhaps communicating with the biosphere. Human mt-DNA contains only 37 genes, while n-DNA has thousands, and it is possible that, over time, n-DNA has been taking on more of the functions of mitochondria, allowing other organelles in the cell to specialize in such activities as protein building, waste elimination, and reproduction.

Eventually, one bacterium engulfed another. The result was that these formerly free organisms now reside within each of your cells. Because of their role in energy metabolism, we might expect larger numbers of mitochondria in the cells of tissues to be more metabolically active. And, indeed, individual cells of the brain, skeletal muscle, heart, kidney, and liver may contain thousands of mitochondria, comprising in some cells up to 40 percent of the cellular material. According to Professor Enzo Nisoli of the University of Milan, a human adult possesses more than ten million billion mitochondria, making up a full 10 percent of the total body weight.

So, while nuclear DNA's main function is to provide the information your cells need to manufacture the various proteins that control the metabolism, repair, and structural integrity of your physical being, it is mitochondrial DNA that directs the production and utilization of your *life energy*. It determines the fate of every cell, tissue, and organ in your body and the energetic fate of your being as a whole.

■ ■ ■

David:
An Energy Crisis

"Where would you like to begin?" I asked "Susan" as I settled into my chair in the examining room.

"Let me tell you. I have a whole list of problems," she began as her mother, who had accompanied her from their home state several hundred miles away, looked on.

"Perfect, because I am a 'whole-listic' doctor," I replied, hoping to lighten her mood.

Susan's problems began about four years earlier, when she had just turned 40. She described her life before becoming ill as active and full. She had actually been quite an accomplished athlete while at the same time working full-time and raising two young children with her husband.

Late in the summer she became suddenly quite ill with what she described as a "bad flu" that pretty much put her out of commission for the greater part of a week. The illness was accompanied by a fever that peaked out at 102 degrees. But it was unlike a normal flu, because after the fever and other symptoms like coughing and diarrhea had passed, she was still experiencing fatigue, even several weeks later.

"I couldn't take it anymore. I just couldn't function," she continued.

Meeting the expectations of her previous active life became insurmountable, so, after a month of waiting it out, she visited her gynecologist, the only physician with whom she had a professional relationship. Blood tests indicated the need for a potent oral antibiotic, which she reluctantly but faithfully took. Two weeks later, Susan's health had not improved.

"Can you describe exactly how you were feeling at that point?" I asked.

She proceeded to list her various complaints, ranging from "brain fog" to fatigue. "I could sleep for ten hours and still wake up tired," she lamented. She went on to describe diffuse aching pain in her muscles and, to a lesser extent, pain in her joints as well.

As is so often the case, Susan began a journey, visiting doctor after doctor who prescribed an extensive battery of medical tests, all of which provided no helpful revelations. She was told on more than one occasion that she should consider seeing a psychiatrist because no explanation was evident in the various physical tests.

"All they did was give her antibiotics and steroids, over and over, and then tell her she was depressed," her mother informed me. The look of frustration on the mother's face rivaled that of her daughter.

About 18 months before I saw Susan, she had visited a doctor in a nearby state who specialized in Lyme disease. Through extensive blood studies, the specialist confirmed that, indeed, Susan was suffering from chronic Lyme disease and prescribed an aggressive antibiotic program that would help her regain her health.

"It was the first glimmer of hope for me," Susan recounted.

She was first placed on two powerful oral antibiotics that she took faithfully for the following six weeks. With no improvement in her condition, she was switched over to intravenous antibiotics after getting an access port installed in her chest to facilitate the administration. Antibiotics were infused intravenously through the port seven days a week for the following four months, but to no avail. Another few rounds of various oral antibiotics were tried, but nothing seemed to help.

By the time Susan came to our center in Naples, Florida, it was very clear that she had almost reached the end of her rope. The desperation in her voice was palpable. Her life was devastated. She was overwhelmed by fatigue, body aches, and a new symptom that had started a year earlier, profound sensitivity to various chemicals. Just passing by a person wearing perfume or aftershave was enough to cause a debilitating headache and even more confusion.

At that point we reviewed the rest of her medical history; aside from a few minor ailments over the years, nothing stood out to provide any meaningful clue to what might be causing this severe condition. Nor did her family history provide any revelatory information. Indeed, her mother confirmed that before the onset of the initial illness, Susan was healthy and enjoying a wonderful relationship with her husband and children.

The standard physical examination added very little insight, with the exception that her blood pressure was a bit low. The neurological examination, which is a more in-depth assessment of various functions of the nervous system, also revealed no abnormalities. Then, as has been my practice for many years, I evaluated her pulse, not in the standard way of counting the beats and checking for a normal rhythm but rather from an Ayurvedic perspective.

Many years ago I was trained in Ayurveda, a system of traditional medicine that dates back to the ancient Vedic period in India. The word *Ayurveda* is derived from the Sanskrit *ayus*, meaning "life," and *veda*, meaning "science" or "knowledge." While I have never considered myself to be a true practitioner of Ayurvedic medicine, nonetheless the pulse diagnosis training has served my patients very well, often providing diagnostic clues when none was otherwise apparent.

And Susan's pulse did tell a story. The Ayurvedic pulse gives information about the three *doshas*, or energies—*vata, pitta,* and *kapha*—that correspond to the energies of wind or air, fire, and earth. The sense I got from Susan's pulse was like a cold wind blowing through a tree that had no leaves to capture and hold the energy. Basically, it felt as if she were "disconnected" from the energy forces blowing through and around her.

I left the examining room and began to review her previous medical reports and laboratory studies—and they were extensive. Interestingly, aside from a very mild anemia, her studies showed nothing to explain her symptoms. Even the blood tests for Lyme disease, which had been repeated several times before, during, and toward the end of her antibiotic treatment, were all normal. Susan and her mother had brought MRI scans, which we reviewed together. Once again, everything looked fine.

When I returned to the examining room, I observed that Susan had displayed all of her numerous nutritional supplements on the examining table. Obviously, along her journey, she had visited a number of complementary medicine practitioners, and each had seemingly given their best advice in hopes of getting her back on her feet.

"Before we go through your supplements," I said, "let me share my thoughts."

I started by giving Susan and her mother an overview of the medical records, including telling them that the Lyme panels were normal, which clearly surprised both of them. I discussed the MRI scans as well as the reports given by the various other practitioners. I then sat back a bit and began to explain my ideas as to why she was so incapacitated.

"I do not have a name for your illness," I said, "but that doesn't mean I can't help you."

I told Susan that the issue ultimately compromising her health was centered on energy. I explained how mitochondria provide energy to the body, and that, for whatever reason, perhaps the initial severe viral infection, her mitochondria were just not fully functional.

"But," I continued, "there is another energy that we need to consider." I explained that energy surrounds every person, that to be alive is to interact with and share in the energy that exists throughout the universe. I carefully watched her face, knowing that this discussion could cause her, or her mother, to feel uncomfortable, but Susan nodded her head with understanding. The really good news was that her mom was also smiling in agreement.

We then went through her various nutritional supplements, and I selected several that would help improve mitochondrial function. I added several more to the regimen as well as coconut oil and DHA, an omega-3 oil. "We're going to get your mitochondria back on line," I explained.

I then went further into the idea of "tapping in" to the energy that surrounds all of us and demonstrated a brief meditation technique that I asked her to perform twice daily.

There wasn't any real need for extensive blood work, because what she had provided was more than comprehensive. But we did check one simple blood test, an evaluation of lipid peroxides that is available at most standard laboratories and provides an assessment of mitochondrial function. It took three weeks to get the results, but what they showed—a very abnormal condition—did confirm that we were on the right track.

After the initial evaluation, we began a series of injections to administer glutathione—a natural compound that enhances mitochondrial function as well as the process of detoxification—in conjunction with the oral supplements.

In addition, I ordered hyperbaric oxygen therapy, a treatment in which Susan sat in a clear acrylic chamber filled with oxygen under pressure. This is the same technology used to help underwater divers recover from decompression sickness caused by returning from pressurized depths to the surface too quickly.

Together, the nutritional supplements, glutathione, and hyperbaric oxygen created a comprehensive program to reestablish mitochondrial health and function in Susan's body. (We will describe each of these in detail later in the book.)

I checked on Susan and her progress during the week that she received her various treatments, then saw her in my office a week later. Even after just one week, Susan was transformed.

But the real evidence was not in how she looked but on her mother's face. I have learned over the years that a parent's concern for an ill child is the same whether the child is 5 or 50. Clearly, Susan's mother had finally seen some daylight at the end of what had been a long tunnel for both of them, and the tears she shed were tears of relief.

"We're going to add a couple more things to your program," I said, recommending some light daily exercises.

Susan eagerly agreed. "I can't believe I'm going to start exercising again," she said, beaming.

In addition to the meditation practice, we began to incorporate affirmations. Several times a day, Susan repeated phrases such as "I am well," and "I am part of all that is around me."

The other new aspect of her program was a day-long fast once every three weeks. Even though she looked puzzled when I first proposed this, I explained both the current science that validates the effects of fasting on mitochondrial function and the rich history of this practice in virtually every one of the world's religions.

Two weeks into the program, Susan was walking 45 minutes each day, was clear-minded enough to keep a journal of her thoughts and activities, and, remarkably, was no longer sensitive to chemicals.

She returned to her home and arranged to receive injections of glutathione three times a week, first at her doctor's office and subsequently with a visiting nurse. She continued the supplement program and fasted every three weeks, as we had discussed. Meditation and affirmations had become a regular part of her day, and she happily reported, "Even my husband is doing them."

We consulted by telephone three weeks after she left our clinic, and she reported that she was able to accompany her husband and two children on bicycle rides. She no longer experienced pain in her muscles, and the headaches and chemical sensitivities had disappeared. I recommended that she reduce the glutathione injections to once a week for the following month.

During our telephone follow-up one month later, Susan reported that all was well. She was continuing with all components of her program and had returned to part-time work. We stopped the intravenous glutathione at that point and made plans to speak several months later.

Our next contact, however, came sooner than that when our office received a Christmas card from Susan and her family that included a photograph of a now-healthy, young-looking woman with her husband and two children.

CHAPTER 5

NEURAL NETWORKS AND HABITS OF THE MIND

Neural networks are unique patterns created by millions of interconnected neurons. Individual neurons extend nerve fibers that reach out to other neurons like the branches on a tree. The links they create can direct traffic along many routes of an extraordinarily intricate web. The neural pathways can join to form networks through which particular patterns of thought, action, and reaction occur. In other words, the neural networks in your brain are made up of a team of nerve cells that have learned to fire together and have subsequently wired together to perform a specific, reproducible function. It is because of neural networks that you are able to accomplish such tasks as chewing gum, snapping your fingers, or recalling the lyrics to "Hey Jude."

CREATION OF YOUR BASIC NEURAL NETWORKS

For the sake of survival, a child needs to develop an instinctive sense for potentially threatening situations. This is why, early in life, we develop aversions and fears in association with events and experiences that, rightly or wrongly, we perceive as dangerous. A great many of these aversions developed while we were still inside our mother's womb.

A flood of stress hormones crosses the placental barrier and informs the fetus of exactly the mood and feeling state that its mother is in. If the mother is happy, the fetus is joyous. If the mother feels safe and loved, this message is registered by the fetus, who also feels safe and loved. If the mother considers terminating the pregnancy, neural networks in the fetal brain are coded for fear as it may intuitively perceive that its life is in danger.

It is in this formative prenatal time that a large percentage of the neural pathways in our limbic brain develop, biasing the way we see and feel the world, and determining our personality. These biases are later reinforced by the codes of conduct and the emotional repertoire that we learned from our parents.

Until about age seven, the human brain is a fertile field, absorbing information, first from the mother's placenta, then from a host of external post-birth influences. Some of these, such as the mother's and father's loving touch and the sound of family laughter, enrich the infant's brain with positive experiences. Other experiences, including that initial inhalation of the first breath, infuse a sense of change, if not danger, in this world outside the mother's warm, watery womb.

During those early years of life, the child's brain is like a digital recorder set on constant record. Or, measured with an electroencephalogram (EEG), the brain-wave frequency of a child from birth to age two is in the delta range, which is also the frequency of the brain waves in a sleeping adult. The brain-wave frequency for a child from two to six is in the theta range, which is what an adult experiences in a state of imagination or reverie or while dreaming. Only into young adulthood does a child's brain become fully adult-functional, operating in the higher frequencies of the alpha or beta wave ranges. In other words, a child under seven years of age basically functions in a hypnotic trance or dream state, which allows that digital recorder in the brain to gather information—*and* form neural pathways—appropriate for the youngster's environment without the filtering and interference of logic and reasoning from the neocortex.

Then, between the ages of 7 and 16, something quite the opposite happens. We take ourselves out of the record mode and start playing around with delete/erase mode instead. During the years of adolescence, our brains eliminate over 80 percent of the interconnections between neurons, in a process known as synaptic pruning.

Why? Because we have learned what's happening in the environment around us. We have a pretty good idea of whom to trust and whom not to trust, who provides food and hugs, and who inflicts pain and punishment. And so we no longer need to gather data from all possible sources, explore behavioral options, and seek alternative ways of experiencing the world.

Shortly after our late teens, we become bound by tradition, anchored by the way things have always been, and entrenched in the belief that everything will remain the same even as the world changes around us. Our worldview is set—not in stone, but in the neural networks of the brain. And while these neural networks communicate chemically and electrically, we experience them as emotions.

THE TYRANNY OF EMOTIONS

There are many schools of thought about emotions, and there is no universally accepted theory or taxonomy of the emotions. Some biologists speak about one set of emotions being instinctual and generated by the amygdala (which is involved in processing the memory of emotional reactions), and another kind as being generated by the prefrontal cortex, and being conscious, cognitive experiences. For the purposes of this book, we will employ these descriptions.

The *cognitive emotions* are conscious, original, and of the moment. It's natural for you to feel happy, angry, or sad at different times in your life, and often for no reason whatsoever. No amount of positive thinking will keep us from occasional unpleasant feelings. Fortunately, these feelings do not last for long. Even though you can have feelings about someone for an entire lifetime, these cognitive emotions are not burdensome, nor do they take up any space in your awareness, and the very act of recollecting them offers you a brief and passing sensation. You might remember your beloved warmly, your childhood sweet-heart lovingly, or the school bully fearfully. These emotions are reasoned and make sense with the situation to which they pertain.

Instinctual emotions are toxic. When you become upset during an argument and remain so long after the exchange is over, it's a sure sign that you're experiencing an instinctual emotion. When overcome with this kind of emotion, you walk around angry without knowing why; your spouse asks you why you were rude to the waiter, and you do not recall being rude; someone stops you to ask you a question, and you nearly bite off their head for no reason at all. When the higher brain functions try to intercede, they are instead hijacked, and you find yourself relentlessly attempting to convince yourself that you were right and the other person was wrong, even years after the event. This results in a refusal to forgive, so that with every recollection of the offending incident, your adrenaline pumps into your nervous system and your body relives the event over and over just as if it were happening again, and you debate how you would have responded differently. Only with diffi-culty—sometimes extreme difficulty—will your nervous system settle down.

Instinctual emotions are produced by ancient survival instincts—often coupled with smoldering memories of trauma—that are wired into our brain. Toxic emotions of fear, sorrow, envy, and anger, which are often passionate, sometimes vio-lent, and always draining, are never experiences of the present moment only. In fact, we can think of them as eruptions caused by trauma that was imprinted into the very fabric of your being. These emotions dredge up stories from your childhood that are super-imposed onto the current moment. They prevent you from expe-riencing authentic feelings, here in the now. Everyone you meet reminds you of someone you have known before, and every new situation seems like a déjà vu. In that way, instinctual emotions are like ancient viral programs that hijack the brain's mainframe and cloud your judgment. And they are the nemesis of true spiritual experience.

Because these emotions are associated with the Four F's—fear, feeding, fighting, and fornicating—they are primitive and instinctual, originating from a prehistoric neurocomputer that we share in common with all mammals. If you experienced physical or verbal abuse in your childhood, you are at risk of associating intimacy with danger in the family you create with your spouse. One terrifying experience during a walk in a big city after nightfall can cause you to link large urban communities with peril. In this way, you rekindle the embers of old memories and bring them into the moment, where they burn with great intensity.

Instinctual emotions linger. If you are angry and it passes after a few minutes, this is a cognitive emotion. If you are angry for 20 days or 20 years, this is an instinctual emotion. Instinctual emotions become like toxic programs that take over our entire neurocomputer. These neural networks cause us to waste precious years in an angry marriage or fettered to an unfulfilling and frustrating job. Eventually, when we think we have finally had enough, we might quit the job or storm out of the marriage, not realizing that what we need to change is our neural networks through which we engage in our current environment and situations.

REINFORCING TOXIC NEURAL PATHWAYS AND SUBCONSCIOUS BELIEFS

Neural networks are a plastic, dynamic architecture, a constellation of neurons that light up momentarily to perform a specific task. This is why, as you mull over a particular thought (good or bad) or practice a particular activity (beneficial or detrimental), you reinforce the neural networks that correlate with those thoughts and skills. Each time a situation reminds you of an actual fearful or dangerous experience from your past and instinctual emotions are brought up, that specific neural network is reinforced. We strengthen the toxic emotions and neural networks in our limbic brain and begin to create subconscious beliefs about life. These beliefs drive our actions and reactions in all experiences.

PTSD, Emotional Stress, and Suffering

When we are exposed to severe trauma, we can develop a condition known as post-traumatic stress disorder (PTSD). Studies show that most people are likely to experience at least one life-threatening or violent event in their lifetime.[1] The studies indicate that even if a person recovers from PTSD, he or she may continue to show mild symptoms.[2] With PTSD many of life's typical events are inappropriately routed through the limbic brain, where we relive, at least from an emotional perspective, the heart-wrenching trauma of events that may have occurred decades ago. PTSD is compounded because the limbic brain, primal as it is, can't tell time and therefore can't distinguish the difference between a painful event that occurred 20 years ago and the memory of that event triggered by a similar situation today.[3] As an example, it was common for soldiers who returned from the Gulf War and the wars in Iraq and Afghanistan to become anxious or distressed when they heard fireworks or other sudden loud noises because their limbic brain did not understand it was no longer in the theater of war. Similarly, couples who go through a bitter divorce may recoil in shock when they hear each other's voice many years after the marriage has ended.

But you do not have to be diagnosed with PTSD to have even seemingly benign events trigger intense emotional reactions.

This reinforcement can be done without our knowledge or when we are milking an emotional *trauma* for sympathy, whether from others or from ourselves. We might say, for example, "I don't have to act maturely; after all, I had a terrible childhood." By creating and repeating such a statement, we reinforce *neural networks* and emotional habits that are as distinct as the postural habits from an old whiplash injury that has affected the vertebra and muscles of the spine. These networks give rise to *emotions,* then *beliefs* that keep us favoring past pain, as well as *behaviors* that continually *reinforce the trauma* as well as the pity we have learned to so successfully milk.

Diagrammed, the pattern looks like this:

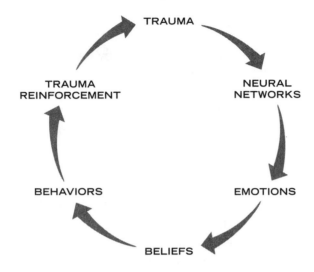

While such a repetitive, circular pattern once served to ensure our survival, it has become toxic and has given rise to erroneous beliefs about the world and acquaintances, friends, and even family. Because beliefs can be unconscious, they may present themselves in ways that surprise us. We may start an intimate relationship that falls apart when we discover the person is not really who we thought he or she was, but the situation might actually be the product of our own unconscious belief that we will never find a partner. Likewise, we may have a terrific career opportunity that collapses because deep down we believe that we are not worthy.

Oddly enough, you can actually reinforce the toxic networks established by traumas by reacting with fear to a *perceived* threat. Unfortunately, whenever a situation is even faintly similar to some painful event from your past, a red flag goes up in your mammalian brain and you perceive it as a possible threat. This is because trauma is not what actually happened but how you stored it as a story in your mind. That is to say, you are impacted by what you *believe* occurred. And this story is kept alive below the threshold of consciousness, without your thinking or being aware.

■ ■ ■

Alberto:
Soul Retrieval

One of my patients was haunted by a recurring image of herself as a six-year-old child when she was hit by an automobile while riding her bicycle. Although "Carol" was unhurt, she remembers lying underneath the stopped vehicle, seeing the underside of the engine, and smelling the overpowering odor of oil and grease. When she recalled this incident, she remembered calling for her mother and father, neither of whom responded. The only one to help her was the stranger who had been driving the automobile.

Years later, Carol continued to be haunted by this feeling of abandonment. She felt that her mother and father had never really been there for her when she needed them and that she could only rely on strangers, who were the very same people who would hurt her. Working with that perception, the neural networks in her limbic brain created erroneous beliefs about friendships and support systems that led her to inappropriate relationships and behaviors.

Carol completely trusted people she met in airplanes and at parties, yet she distrusted her family and friends who genuinely tried to advise and help her. She felt tremendous anger toward her parents but would forgive strangers for the most heinous acts.

Carol only began to heal when I helped her revisit that event during a guided meditation. We coaxed that part of her personality that had "split off" or disassociated during the accident to come back. In doing so, we had to reassure Little Carol that Big Carol would look after her and protect her and welcome her with gifts and beauty. Shamans refer to this process as *soul retrieval,* and, in effect, I did help Carol recover lost qualities of her soul: trust, curiosity, security, confidence, and spontaneity. As she embraced these qualities, she opened the way for new neural pathways that would allow her to experience the world more creatively. She began to perceive people and situations in a new way, seeing opportunities where before she had only seen adversity.

■ ■ ■

ENDING THE PROPENSITY FOR SUFFERING

For many years, psychology embraced the idea that destructive emotions could be repaired with therapy, a view that is questioned today by some practitioners, who are even debating the legitimacy of psychology itself. The psychoanalyst James Hillman, for example, writes, "The failure of psychotherapy to make clear its legitimacy has resulted in psychologies which are bastard sciences and degenerate philosophies. Psychotherapy has attempted to support its pedigree by appropriating logics unsuited for investigating its area. As these borrowed methods fail one by one, psychotherapy seems more and more dubious—neither good physics, good philosophy, nor good religion."[4] In our respective professions, we (the authors) have come to know many dedicated psychotherapists who are working in schools, prisons, and neighborhood health centers. These practitioners are fiercely committed to helping their patients alleviate their suffering and fit better into society. Yet, we agree that popular psychological platitudes and pop spirituality have served little purpose beyond miring us further in our painful stories.

While the media have popularized issues regarding inadequate parents, abandonment, and low self-esteem, commentators and critics have fallen far short of providing satisfying explanations that will console our complex personalities. At best, media attention and open dialogue have helped many of us understand how the painful events and trauma we experienced in childhood have shaped our relationships. Yet, this understanding has done little to rewire the neural networks in our brain that keep us trapped in these stories, which is the only thing that could really help us feel better about ourselves or free us to lead more fulfilling lives.

Instead, we go around explaining to ourselves and others why we're incapable of loving or trusting, or why we are reluctant to believe in our self-worth. We claim it is because our mothers didn't nurture us or our fathers mistreated us. In other words, we continue to subscribe to debilitating narratives—many of them of our own creation—about who we are and what we are capable of accomplishing. And we keep buying self-help titles that perennially top the best-seller lists!

So, why don't we get better? Because we are looking for answers in all the wrong places.

■ ■ ■

Alberto:
Gaining Respect for Self

A patient, "Chris," once said to me, "Every job I've had has been stressful because I inevitably end up with a tyrannical boss who doesn't respect my talent or contributions." This man had been in psychotherapy for many years, trying to understand why he "got no respect." He had exhaustively dissected his family dynamics and had worked very hard to uncover the reasons why he kept repeating this self-defeating pattern in his professional life.

I carefully pointed out to him that the answer lay in the neural networks of his brain that made sure familiar "reality" kept repeating itself. Psychology had helped him understand the childhood trauma that had established these networks in the first place—the fact that he was the eldest child of an elderly father, that he was seldom included by playmates when they chose teams, that he was driven to become an overachiever in school, and that he later dropped out of school altogether. But his understanding of the origins of his conflict with his bosses did not result in better everyday relationships, just as understanding how a virus affects the immune system does not cure the flu. I recommended brain-enriching nutrients, knowing these would help regions in his limbic brain heal, which would allow new, higher cortical pathways to be established through other methods I would provide.

I also assigned Chris the contemplative practice of sitting quietly for ten minutes every morning and counting his breaths. I told him to ask himself, "Who am I?" and to discard every answer that came to him. One morning, in a sudden moment of insight, Chris realized that the people he worked for were not "demanding" of him or "demeaning" him as he had thought; rather, they simply expected the best from him because they saw a potential that he himself had not yet been able—or ready—to recognize.

My work with Chris then consisted of crafting a map for his future that would guide him to new beliefs, new behaviors, and a new direction in life founded on a deep and trusting relationship with the world.

■ ■ ■

The Seven Deadly Sins

In early Christian times, many people feared being consumed by the Seven Deadly Sins: wrath, greed, lust, sloth, envy, gluttony, and pride. These instinctual emotions were recognized as being so powerful that Peter Binsfeld, a 16th-century German theologian and bishop, attributed each one of these sins to a particular demon: Satan (wrath), Mammon (greed), Asmodeus (lust), Belphegor (sloth), Leviathan (envy), Beelzebub (gluttony), and Lucifer (pride). He explained his theory in his influential book, *De confessionibus maleficarum et sagarum* (Of the Confessions of Warlocks and Witches). Had Bishop Binsfeld been not so inclined toward a purely demonic analysis of human error and more versed in the anatomy of the brain, he might have come up with a more scientific message instead of blaming human "sins" on such a hellishly colorful cast of characters. Alas, the study of the brain's physical anatomy through dissection was not possible at that time because, without preservation, the brain turns to the consistency of a milkshake a few hours after death.

Yet, Bishop Binsfeld, a relative moderate who, unlike other inquisitors, believed children should not be burned at the stake, was not far off the mark when he claimed that demons can tempt humans away from a life of grace and into eternal damnation. You see, while inquisitional wisdom, such as it was, believed that demons seduced humans with lust, greed, gluttony, wrath, envy, sloth, and pride, these human "weaknesses" actually arise from ancient and outdated programs in the limbic brain.

CHAPTER 6

HOW STRESS HARMS THE BRAIN

From an engineering standpoint, stress can be defined as the amount of resistance a material offers to being reshaped and reformed. When you place a load on a steel beam, the beam resists, keeping the building from collapsing. If the load is great enough, the beam gives way and the structure suffers damage or collapses. Psychological stress is similar. When we can no longer resist forces that are trying to shape and mold us, whether they are our spouse's behavior or our nation's economic decline, we break down, becoming anxious and depressed, unable to cope.

SOCIETAL AND ENVIRONMENTAL STRESS

Sources of stress are everywhere. The rate of technological change has never been as accelerated as it is today. College students are training for jobs that don't yet exist. Americans in the workforce today can expect to go through at least three career changes in the course of their professional lives. Even thinking about this is stressful.

And while societal stressors affect our emotional health, bio-chemical stressors are also wreaking havoc inside our bodies. For example, many pesticides kill insects by destroying mitochondrial function, thus raising the obvious question: could pesticides contribute to the development of Parkinson's in the general population? The answer has proved to be a resounding yes, with studies, beginning in 2000, showing a significant increase in the risk of developing Parkinson's from even casual use of pesticides such as rotenone. Joan Stephenson, Ph.D., reported in the widely respected *Journal of the American Medical Association,* "Handling or applying insecticides also was linked with significantly elevated rates of Parkinson's disease. Those who used insecticides in the garden showed a 50 percent increased risk of the disorder compared with those who had never been exposed to home pesticides of any type. In-home use of insect-killing chemicals was associated with a 70 percent increased risk of Parkinson's disease, compared with no use of pesticide."[1] And since pesticides directly target mitochondrial function, there's reason for much broader concern as mitochondrial function is impaired in all manner of neurodegenerative diseases, including Alzheimer's, multiple sclerosis, autism, and epilepsy. And new research is focusing on the damaging effects on mitochondrial function as an explanation of the significant increase in risk for diabetes in people exposed to pesticides.

And environmental toxins don't just affect individuals directly; their effects are transmitted to the next generation. Recent blood tests taken from the umbilical cords of newborns in the United States and Europe showed contamination by more than 200 toxic chemicals, including plastics.[2] These babies are being born with a tremendous toxic burden that may greatly increase their chances of developing serious illnesses and degenerative brain disorders later in life.

And while these infants have no say in what toxins their mothers may have consumed, willingly or inadvertently, consenting adults are choosing to allow known toxins to enter their bodies. For example, it's common knowledge that mercury fillings used by dentists release toxic gases that are readily absorbed by fat in the brain, where they interfere with the functioning of the nervous system. Unfortunately, it's very difficult to get this mercury poisoning out of the body

Whether transmitted in utero, ingested, inhaled, absorbed through the skin, or drilled into our teeth, such toxins impact our cells, which were not designed to eliminate large quantities of harmful environmental poisons.

ACUTE AND CHRONIC STRESS

Psychologists identify two kinds of stress: acute and chronic. Both affect the health of mitochondria in our cells and our general well-being.

Acute stress is relatively short-lived. It's what you encounter when faced with a novel learning situation, and it is actually good for you in the sense that it allows you to remember the event, be it positive or negative. This is the type of stress you experience when you're challenged to be your best, whether as a child about to make your first solo musical performance at school or as an adult when faced with a demanding intellectual situation or a physical challenge such as running a marathon. I (Alberto) was in Chile during the devastating 8.8 magnitude earthquake of 2010. While it was a terrifying experience to have the earth move under my feet for several minutes, this catastrophe brought out the best in people, as neighbors rallied to help each other tend to those who were hurt and to help rebuild their homes and their lives.

Chronic stress is long-lasting. It occurs when you worry all month about how you're going to make your mortgage payment, or when you dread every day waking up next to the person you married many years earlier, or when your cells are continuously burdened with eliminating toxic wastes and heavy metals acquired from a polluted environment and now stored within the cell wall. The great earthquake in Chile was followed by a month of aftershocks—more than 300 greater than 5.0 in magnitude in total. During this month, everyone slept fitfully, as they did not know when the earth would start shaking again. After two weeks, the entire population was sleep-deprived and exhausted, with their fight-or-flight systems stuck in the on position because there was no one to fight and nowhere to flee.

Our bodies have a system in place to deal with stress. The HPA axis—which refers to three organs, the hypothalamus, the pituitary, and the adrenal glands—regulates our fight-or-flight system. The pituitary gland and hypothalamus are both located within the limbic brain, and the adrenal glands are located above the kidneys. If the amygdala perceives an imminent threat, the HPA axis, rather than passing the signal along to the neocortex for logical processing, releases stress hormones—cortisol and adrenaline—into the bloodstream. These steroids give us quick energy, increase our heart rate, direct blood away from digestion and other non-emergency body functions, and reroute blood to our extremities and muscles so we can fight or flee. The advantages offered by the rapid response of our HPA axis are clear. Just as primitive man was able to avoid being attacked by an animal during a hunt, we today can quickly move out of the way of an oncoming car or an angry colleague.

In times of danger, this chemical influx is necessary to help us fight or flee, but we can get locked into a state of chronic stress when the adrenal glands don't receive a signal to stop producing these hormones. Unlike acute stress, which serves a positive purpose, chronic stress is very destructive. In Colonial times the legendary pirates of the Caribbean learned that citizens in a city under siege were more effectively worn down by the sound of cannons firing than by the actual damage done to their town by the cannonballs. This was because the sounds of the guns kept the townspeople in a state of chronic stress, unable to fight or flee, or get a good night's rest. Long-term exposure to stress has very profound consequences.

THE DETRIMENTAL EFFECTS OF CHRONIC STRESS

Relating this information back to what we have already learned about the evolution of the brain, it's important to note that the stress hormone cortisol, which is produced in excessive amounts when the HPA axis is locked in a state of chronic stress, increases the damaging effects of free radicals in the neurons of the hippocampus. This causes damage to the mitochondria, which in turn causes even more free radical production. The final act in this tragic play is that the hippocampal neurons themselves perish through the process of apoptosis. And when hippocampal neurons die, learning and creativity become almost impossible. And brain synergy is out of the question. The avoidance of pain overshadows natural curiosity; we hesitate to rock the boat; we hoard needlessly and risk foolishly. We become paralyzed by an inability to discover novel solutions and are unable to *think* or *feel* originally anymore. If we remain under acute stress long enough, our adrenals eventually give out and we become drained and exhausted.

In a recent study, Eduardo Dias-Ferreira and his colleagues at the University of Minho in Braga, Portugal, demonstrated that chronically stressed rats lose their ability to break out of repetitive behavior patterns and become less creative and less cunning.[3] Essentially, stress changes the rodents' behavior, predisposing the animals to doing the same things over and over. In commenting on the study, Robert Sapolsky a neurobiologist who studies stress at Stanford University School of Medicine, remarked, "This is a great model for understanding why we end up in a rut, and then dig ourselves deeper and deeper into that rut . . . we're lousy at recognizing when our normal coping mechanisms aren't working."[4]

Chronic stress can lead to a rut in which the wiring of our neural networks keeps us repeating the same dysfunctional behavior and hoping for a different outcome. As we experience depression and repetitive behaviors that stem from chronic stress, we're less capable of analytic thought. The stress hormones released into the bloodstream keep us at a lower order of brain function, unable to attain synergy. Like iron and carbon, we remain brittle and easily afflicted, unable to find the strength of steel. We find it increasingly difficult to learn from past experiences, to alter the beliefs that cause us to re-create those experiences again and again, and to break out of our behavioral ruts. Because of the way our brains have been wired by stress and trauma, we're unable to think or feel our way out of personal crises.

Dr. Sapolsky, in his book *Stress, the Aging Brain, and the Mechanisms of Neuron Death,* eloquently describes the science that correlates stress, exposure to cortisol, and the ultimate destruction of the hippocampus. His extensive research with rodents and primates clearly supports the contention that this stress-induced neuro-degenerative process also occurs in humans. Interestingly, Sapolsky points out that elevated cortisol levels are found in at least 50 percent of Alzheimer's patients.[5]

Fortunately, in the last several years, researchers have discovered that we can stop this cascade of destructive chemical events. Research using animals has shown that an elevated level of brain-derived neurotrophic factor (BDNF), which is a protective brain hormone increased by such activities as calorie reduction, fasting, and mental and physical exercise, imparts a high level of protection for the hippocampus, making it resistant to damage from elevated cortisol; and we now understand that in humans, BDNF plays the identical role.

■ ■ ■

Alberto:
Lifting the Dark Cloud

"Natasha" came to see me complaining that she was very unhappy with her life and her marriage. She and her husband had three young children, and she felt her life had been reduced to being a soccer mom. Before having her children, she had been a designer for a popular magazine, but now felt her life was direc-tionless. She thought herself to be mildly depressed and was con-sidering going on medication to treat her changing moods.

One of the tenets of shamanic energy medicine is that nothing is only what it seems to be. I asked Natasha if she was taking medi-cation, and she explained that she was taking medicine for her thyroid. I entered the quiet state of awareness that facilitates the shaman's "seeing" and began to scan Natasha's Luminous Energy Field, looking for pools of stagnant energy that might indicate pathology. I also checked her chakras, the energy centers along the spine.

The chakras are swirling vortexes of energy, shaped like a funnel. The large end of the funnel extends a couple of inches outside the skin, while the narrow end connects to the spinal cord and the endocrine glands that produce hormones and release them into the bloodstream. Hindu texts describe chakras as spinning vortexes of energy, and sages in the Americas identify them as "wells of light." My own investigation showed me that the chakras coincide with the nerve plexuses, that is, networks of intersecting nerves.

I noticed that Natasha's throat chakra was spinning sluggishly, which was not surprising, since her thyroid was hypoactive. Then I noticed that her sixth chakra, located at the forehead, was withered and completely shut down like some flower that had closed its petals a long time ago. The sixth chakra is connected to the pituitary gland, the *P* in the HPA axis.

As I continued to scan Natasha's Luminous Energy Field, I observed that there was no physical pathology, which generally appears as pools of dark, stagnant energy that settle over an organ or tissue. Instead, I saw the markings of emotional trauma, which appear as ribbons of various luminous colors swirling around the field and interfering with the chakras. These are manifestations of toxic neural networks and are always an indication of early life trauma.

I asked Natasha what happened to her when she was six or seven years of age, and she explained that she and her family were living in the Bryansk region of Russia, close to the Chernobyl nuclear power plant, when reactor number four exploded in 1986. This explosion deposited radioactive iodine in the fields and pastures surrounding Chernobyl, which caused the evacuation of more than 200,000 people, including Natasha's family. This forced mass exodus proved to be a very traumatic and disruptive event in their lives because they knew they would never return to their homes.

Because iodine binds to the thyroid, Natasha's story might explain her thyroid condition. But even though she had not suffered any further radiation exposure and lived in Canada, where her doctors monitored her closely, she still suffered from trauma and fear caused by this nuclear explosion.

In my training as a shaman, I had learned to track and intervene at the level of my client's energetic matrix, a practice that we at the Healing the Light Body School teach our students to do with great success. I was able to clear these ribbons of noxious energy, breaking up the habitual patterns through which Natasha perceived the world and allowing her to grow new neural networks in her brain.

I also "tuned up" her second chakra, which is connected to the adrenals, getting it to spin in harmony with the rest of her energy system. And I reset her fight-or-flight system using an energy intervention practiced by shamans and described in my book *Shaman, Healer, Sage.* This was necessary because her HPA axis had been on high alert since she was six, exhausting her adrenals and throwing off her entire hormonal system.

But I also knew that, until Natasha repaired her hippocampus, she would not be able to heal from the memory of trauma and loss she suffered as a child. I asked Natasha to start taking DHA daily and to eliminate all stimulants such as coffee from her diet. And I advised her to practice the shamanic meditations.

Three months later, the dark cloud began to lift from Natasha's body. She had found a part-time job with a local magazine, and her family life had improved dramatically.

■ ■ ■

CHANGING THE HIPPOCAMPUS SET POINT

To protect against the damage of chronic stress is to change the hippocampus set point. As research continued to expose the connection between cortisol production and hippocampal damage, scientists began to wonder what actually controlled the amount of cortisol produced by the adrenal glands during a stressful event. It has long been recognized, for example, that not only do older humans and animals alike generally have higher levels of cortisol, but the degree of cortisol production following stress also seems to increase with age. Great efforts have been made to find the "pacemaker" for the adrenal gland. Scientists reasoned that if such a structure indeed existed in the human body, perhaps there is also a way to control excess cortisol production. In this way, the damage to the hippocampus that occurs during normal aging—and at a much faster rate in Alzheimer's patients—could be reduced.

Much to the surprise of many, the ultimate governor of adrenal activity is none other than the hippocampus itself. That's right; the hippocampus actually regulates the adrenal's production of cortisol, in effect controlling its own fate! When functioning optimally, the hippocampus is able to maintain cortisol production in response to stress at a normal level. However, when the hippocampus is damaged, it loses this ability and calls for excessive cortisol production.

To understand what it means to reset your hippocampal set point, think of the hippocampus as being like the thermostat in your home. With stress and trauma, the set point of the hippocampus changes, much as when you adjust the temperature on your air conditioner. Lowering the thermostat makes the air conditioner run longer: lowering the set point of the hippocampus has the same effect on the adrenals.

We now understand that the hippocampus set point that modulates the adrenal's production of cortisol is programmed very early in life. Thus, trauma at a young age increases the hippocampus's sensitivity to cortisol. And this sets the stage for an ever-increasing decline in hippocampal function in adulthood, which inhibits our ability to respond to situations in novel ways.

Researchers have wondered if intervention could perhaps lower cortisol levels. If stress raised cortisol, they reasoned, then perhaps living a nonstressful life could lower it. The pioneering work in this area was carried out by the late psychoneuroendocrinologist Seymour "Gig" Levine, beginning in 1962. His groundbreaking research demonstrated that when laboratory guinea pigs were lovingly handled as pups, their cortisol secretion was diminished and this reduction persisted into adulthood.

Levine's early experiments paved the way for countless other researchers who tested a variety of animals, including primates, to reaffirm that positive emotional experiences can provide protection to the delicate hippocampus by reducing cortisol production. While the set point of hippocampal control of adrenal cortisol production may be genetically determined, we now understand that all positive and negative life experiences, whether in childhood or adulthood, can reset that sensitivity.

So we need not run off to a secluded cabin in the woods to ensure a stress-free life, appealing as this may be. For, as many of us have discovered, we take our ghosts and demons with us wherever we go, and our dramas become like the story of the traveler who meets a fellow traveler on the road, going the opposite direction, and asks him what the people were like in the city he is going to. The first traveler responds by asking him what the people were like in the city he just left. "It was full of thieves and liars. There was not a decent person in the town," he states. To which the other traveler replies, "It will be exactly the same in the next town."

The ongoing biochemical assault from stress hormones on our hippocampus makes it impossible to heal from emotional trauma. Like the second traveler above, everywhere we go seems to be populated by liars and thieves. But this can also be a beneficial signal. When we feel imprisoned by our toxic emotions, we *know* at some core level that we must heal our lifelong trauma. We *know* that in order to regain our sanity and discover new behaviors, we must change.

While the destructive emotions associated with past traumas, whether real or imagined, may tend to dominate your moods, you are nevertheless capable of developing neural networks that allow you to think and feel differently. You have the ability to experience events without letting the past cast them in a negative light. Once the limbic brain is enlisted to serve the greater brain synergy, you begin to establish new neural networks for joy, well-being, and creativity.

■ ■ ■

David:
The Greatest Thing

In the spring of 2001, I had the opportunity to present a lecture titled "Stress, Aging, and Neurodegenerative Disorders" at the International Symposium on Functional Medicine in Vancouver, British Columbia. During my presentation, I explained to the physicians and researchers the concepts of stress, the hippocampus, and resetting the hippocampus set point, as described above, using various technical slides and animations to help clarify the relationship between stress and actual functional loss in the brain.

As I was doing so, it became clear to me that most of the research, and even most of my slides, focused on the negative—that stress is bad news. But I wanted to share the good news, too—that positive emotion can heal the brain. So I chose to end the presentation with a slide that showed a photograph of my daughter, perhaps four months old at the time, sleeping peacefully on my wife's chest. I included an audio clip of Nat King Cole's song "Nature Boy," in which he sings about the importance of learning how to love and accept love in return.

■ ■ ■

THE POSITIVES OF STRESS

But we must remember that stress isn't all bad. In fact, it is essential for all human progress, just as necessity is the mother of invention. When we are unable to respond with creativity to a challenging situation, it is because we are caught in a neural rut. Our brain's wiring won't permit it. When you go to the gym for strength training, you put stress on your muscles, and at the end of the workout, you leave with a toned body and a feeling of accomplishment. Biological stress on a species, such as that caused by a change in food availability due to long-term drought, is resolved through creative coping or adapting. Without the stress of a changing ecosystem, our apelike ancestors would never have left the savannas of Africa for more fertile areas in Asia and Europe; they would not have started walking on two legs instead of four. In those cases, stress was nature's way of inviting the wisest and most adaptable to survive.

At our present point in human history, with a changing eco-system and an increased toxic load from poisons in our food and water, our species is once again faced with the challenge of long-term survival. And the enlightenment required of us may be no less daunting than having to learn to walk upright on two legs.

CHAPTER 7

THE GIFT OF NEUROPLASTICITY

Although we originally developed our amygdala-based fight-or-flight response and our instinctual emotions in order to ensure our survival as a species, allowing the amygdala to control our brain can result, as we've seen, in a virtually crippling situation in which our survival is actually compromised.

Luckily, the human brain has the ability to rewire itself and form new connections between neurons so that we do not continue playing over again the tired primitive programs of aggression and fear. Only recently have researchers discovered the potential of the human brain and come to truly appreciate the positive implications of neuroplasticity—the brain's ability to create new neural networks—for both our individual health as well as for society in general.

We now understand how to harness our brain's neuroplasticity to enhance certain neural pathways. In essence, we can alter our brain function so that we can more fully access those areas that pave the way for freedom from trauma and destructive emotions; this also allows us to express the genes for health and longevity and even enlightenment.

Neuroscientists have come a long way over the past 25 years. They have replaced the once-accepted paradigm of the brain as a hardwired, fixed, and immutable organ with the belief in neuroplasticity, which celebrates its dynamic ability to learn, adapt, and change.

■ ■ ■

David:
A Shift in My Understanding

When I was young, I didn't have the opportunity to spend much time with my father because he maintained a very busy practice in neurosurgery in south Florida. Clearly, he too recognized this shortcoming in our relationship, and one day he came up with a solution: he invited me to the operating room to watch him remove a tumor from the base of a patient's brain. What a way to spend a Saturday afternoon, especially considering that I was a young teenager at the time! I soon made these visits to the operating room a regular part of my weekends. In retrospect, I believe my dad even made the effort to schedule surgery on Saturdays so I could join him. And, of course, he taught me the proper procedures to maintain a sterile operating room. These procedures would take many hours, so, to pass the time, my father would explain the specific function of that part of the brain upon which we were operating. "This area," he would say, for example, "is called Broca's Area, named for Pierre-Paul Broca, a French fellow who, back in 1861, determined that this area controlled speech." Over time, he described the entire brain in detail, always weaving some bit of historical color into the description.

These experiences at a very impressionable age provided me with a rich and expansive understanding of neuroscience. Later, the idea that specific parts of the brain were dedicated to specific functions was reinforced by the brain research I pursued in college, and it was also one of the key themes in my early publications in the *Journal of Neurosurgery*. Medical school further stressed this connection between particular functions and specific parts of the brain. Hearing of this relationship from so many sources, including my dad, certainly demonstrated that this mentality was pervasive throughout the medical field. And this concept was further reinforced during my years of neurology training. Indeed, it was often said that neurologists learned functional brain anatomy "stroke by stroke." That is to say, whenever a patient was admitted to the hospital with a stroke in a particular area of the brain, neurologists would note the physical disability that correlated with it and thereby identified which function the damaged brain area served.

This simple mechanical structure/function relationship began to unravel, at least for me, in the late 1980s, when I began to note that some patients would regain considerable function of a particular area of the body following a stroke, even though there had been no observable change in their brain imaging studies. So, while a patient's MRI continued to show damage in, for example, the part of the brain that controls the left hand, not infrequently the brain would somehow "heal" and functionality of the left hand would return. As more and more neurologists, therapists, and patients observed this unusual phenomenon, neuroscientists began to offer explanations that contradicted the prevailing view of the brain's abilities.

To this day, I vividly recall what would later become a turning point for me in my understanding of the brain. "Michael," a 58-year-old graphic designer from North Carolina, came to see me in 1988. He reported that 14 months prior to his visit he suddenly became unable to speak. "I knew what I wanted to say, but I just couldn't produce the words," he recounted with perfect fluency. My first thought was that he had experienced a transient ischemic attack (TIA), characterized by a brief decline in blood supply to a particular region of the brain—in this case, an area associated with language expression. But, as he continued, he revealed that his speech had been compromised for at least six months following the attack. There was nothing "transient" about it. And while his recovery had been profound, clearly he wanted to do everything he could to prevent any further brain events.

We reviewed an MRI scan of his brain that had been taken just two months prior to his visit at our clinic, and there, for all to see, was evidence of severe damage and loss of tissue, not only in the area associated with speech, but also in the adjacent areas associated with facial movement and control of the right arm. Nonetheless, his examination revealed no deficits whatsoever. What had happened? Clearly, his brain hadn't "healed"—at least not physically—because the area of his initial stroke was still damaged, according to the MRI. Yet, his brain had *adapted;* that is, it had begun to use *alternative pathways* to regain functionality of the related affected part of his body.

Of course, the accepted paradigm at the time considered this concept fanciful. Now, however, we know that the brain does have the ability to change and reorganize itself in regard to the functions it performs. This process is called neuroplasticity, and it is a gift on par with neurogenesis, the brain's ability to generate new cells throughout our lifetimes.

■ ■ ■

CHANGING OUR NEURAL NETWORKS

Through neuroplasticity the brain is able to rewire neural pathways, and even establish new neural superhighways. When a person suffers a stroke and loses function in the right hand, for example, the brain can create new pathways that may allow the left hand to perform some of the functions previously done only by the right.

Neural networks are created by focused, engaged stimulation. It takes more than simple repetition to create neural networks. Professional athletes have long known that practice does not necessarily make perfect, because bad practice simply reinforces a less than ideal pathway in the brain. Likewise, repeating a prayer over and over without positive focused intention makes enlightenment less likely. If you want to experiment, try brushing your teeth or holding your fork with your nondominant hand and notice how much concentration is required to perform this simple task. Likewise, the practice of joy, kindness, and forgiveness take focused attention to develop, but the more you exercise them, the more easily and naturally they come.

Michael Merzenich, professor emeritus at the University of California, San Francisco, performed a series of experiments in the mid-1990s that demonstrate the need for focused attention in order to learn new skills and behaviors. In one experiment, he applied a tapping stimulus to the fingers of two groups of monkeys. When the rhythm of the tapping occasionally changed, monkeys in one group received a reward of juice for responding to the change. The other group of monkeys was not rewarded for responding. After six weeks, Merzenich examined the monkeys' brains. The animals who had paid close attention to the stimulus, waiting for the change in rhythm so they could collect their reward, exhibited profound differences in the areas of the brain associated with processing tactile stimuli. No such changes were seen in the brains of the monkeys who were not rewarded for paying attention to the stimulus even though the stimulus, the tapping on their fingers, was exactly the same for both groups.[1]

This is another reason why all those pats on the back, gold stars, recognition ribbons, and colorful merit badges we earned as children are so important to the brain! Even if those once-cherished prizes are now collecting dust on a shelf or stored in a forgotten box in the closet, the brain still remembers and appreciates the positive reinforcement from that impressionable time.

As Merzenich pointed out, the choices you make actually do influence the physical structures, the neural networks, in your brain. He remarked, "Experience coupled with attention leads to physical changes in the structure and future functioning of the nervous system. This leaves us with a clear physiological fact . . . moment by moment we choose and sculpt how our ever-changing minds will work, we choose who we will be the next moment in a very real sense, and these choices are left embossed in physical form on our material selves."[2]

The need for focused attention is further affirmed by Joe Dispenza in his book *Evolve Your Brain*: "The key ingredient in making these neural connections . . . is focused attention. When we mentally attend to whatever we are learning, the brain can map the information on which we are focusing. On the other hand, when we don't pay complete attention to what we are doing in the present moment, our brain activates a host of other synaptic networks that can distract it from its original intention. Without focused concentration, brain connections are not made, and memory is not stored."[3]

So, attention matters, whether it is gentle meditation or the intense concentration of an athlete at a critical competitive moment. As Sharon Begley, an award-winning science writer summarized in a *Wall Street Journal* article in 2007: "The discovery that neuroplasticity cannot occur without attention has important implications. If a skill becomes so routine you can do it on autopilot, practicing it will no longer change the brain. And if you take up mental exercises to keep your brain young, they will not be as effective if you become able to do them without paying much attention."[4]

OVERCOMING TOXIC EMOTIONS

Sensing and responding to threats instinctively through our emotions is one role of the limbic brain, which enables us to develop behaviors that keep us out of harm's way. Just as our ancestors learned during our hunter-gatherer past that danger lurked in a particular part of the forest and that it wasn't safe to stray away from our clan, so we too are taught to "stop, look, listen" before crossing a street, through which we gain a deep respect for danger from oncoming vehicles. The problem in responding instinctively to all perceived threats is that we turn over to our amygdala control of our responses rather than using the logic of the prefrontal cortex.

With our new understanding of neuroplasticity, we know that our brain can adapt not only to injuries but, more importantly, in response to any and all experiences we may encounter. This frees us from merely responding reflexively as a consequence of genetically determined hardwiring. Alvaro Pascual-Leone, a neurology researcher at Harvard Medical School, recently stated that neuroplasticity "is an intrinsic property of the human brain and represents evolution's invention to enable the nervous system to escape the restrictions of its own genome and thus adapt to environmental pressures, physiologic changes, and experiences."[5]

Researchers have discovered that not only can we create new neural networks, but also we can create them to be powerful enough to overcome our instinctive emotional reactions. In an experiment, individuals were asked to do two tasks—one perceptual and one intellectual. The first task was to match the emotion of anger or fear that was apparent in images of faces projected onto a screen—a perceptual task involving images. They were then asked to look at the faces and associate them with the words *anger* or *fear*—an intellectual task involving words. When matching the angry or frightened expression, participants experienced increased blood flow to the amygdala, the primary fear center of the brain. In contrast, when the participants assigned the word labels to the image, blood flow to the amygdala diminished while circulation to the right prefrontal cortex increased. Because the prefrontal region is associated with overriding our primitive emotional responses, the researchers concluded that we can develop new neural networks in higher regions of the brain and reduce these responses.

The neural networks formed while in our mother's womb and during childhood are the foundation for our later beliefs. They are the beliefs we carry into adulthood and through which we understand and interpret our experiences. And while the first lessons from our infancy generally serve us well, they can negatively color future experiences that would otherwise have been perceived as benign or even positive.

The science of neuroplasticity suggests that you can rewire the circuits of the brain and create new, more positive associations within your day-to-day experiences. Shamans learned that the instinctual survival emotions of fear, lust, and anger that color the way you respond to the events of your life are actually the causes of illness. You no longer have to succumb to the tyranny of the emotional limbic brain with its self-created nightmares that prevent you from experiencing joy. You don't have to experience fearful responses when faced with new situations. Instead, you can come to them fresh, open to the possibilities they present.

You can change the sounding board by which you judge your present experience and allow yourself to see the world, quite literally, in a new light. You can set aside the old trauma and drama, and become enlightened to what blinded you before, awakened to what is new, exciting, rich, prosperous, healthy, and joyful.

To free yourself from the immediate emotional responses of the limbic brain, you must accomplish two tasks. First, you have to enhance your brain's physiology, which you can achieve by making specific dietary and lifestyle modifications. Second, once your brain has been optimized, you can take full advantage of its powerful ability to develop pathways that will enable you to experience people and events you once perceived as negative, instead, as enriching, fulfilling, and positive.

■ ■ ■

Alberto:
Men with Beards

I grew up in Cuba during the Communist revolution and witnessed the aftermath of tremendous violence: An old woman hosing off what looked like fresh blood on her driveway. Militiamen storming through our front door, demanding to know where my father was, threatening to hurt my mother. For years, I was unable to trust people, especially anyone who sported a beard, because all the militiamen, after years of fighting in the mountains, were bearded.

Shortly after we arrived in the United States, Woodstock, the Summer of Love, and the hippie era started, and all my male friends let their hair down and grew a beard! Immediately, after the first hairs appeared on their faces, I found myself shying away from their friendship even though I had also let my hair grow long. All my friends would ask me why I was clean-shaven. I understood perfectly well why I was reacting in this manner, yet I was not able to change my reaction. The neural networks in my limbic brain kept superimposing the images of violence from my childhood onto the peaceniks and flower children!

■ ■ ■

THE MECHANICS OF NEUROPLASTICITY

Michael was able to regain the use of his speech because his brain established new neural pathways that, fortunately for him, allowed for the dramatic return of function. But how do individual neurons actually connect? What initiates the connection and keeps them connected?

While the individual working unit of the brain is the single neuron, even simple tasks require that vast numbers of interconnected neurons function as a unit or network devoted to accomplishing even the simplest activity. Joe Dispenza, in his book *Evolve Your Brain,* eloquently described a neural network as "literally millions of neurons firing together in diverse compartments, modules, sections, and subregions throughout the entire brain. They team up to form communities of nerve cells that act in unison as a group, clustered together in relation to a particular concept, idea, memory, skill, or habit. Whole patterns of neurons throughout the brain become connected through the process of learning, to produce a unique level of mind."[6]

Pioneering research into neuroplasticity dates back to the work of Canadian psychologist Donald Hebb, who proposed a theory of what he called "cell assembly" to explain how neurons develop a relationship with one another. In his landmark book, *The Organization of Behavior,* published in 1949, Dr. Hebb hypothesized that "neurons that fire together, wire together," which is commonly referred to as Hebb's law.

While the precise biochemical changes that take place to facilitate this growth process when neurons connect to form neural networks is quite complex, researchers generally agree that brain-derived neurotrophic factor (BDNF) creates the fertile ground for this union to take place, helping transform a mere embrace of two neurons into an eternal dance.

The corollary of Dr. Hebb's "neurons that fire together, wire together" hypothesis is that patterned thoughts and activities must be maintained if the neural networks associated with those activities are to remain functional. Or, in complementary terms: neurons that don't fire together don't remain wired together.

So, is the glass half full or is it half empty? It's both.

And is that good news or bad news? Thankfully, it's all good news.

The good news is that, with focused attention, as stated earlier, you can change your thoughts, change your activities, and change your behaviors to make a positive improvement in your life. The other good news is that if you don't reinforce the neural networks currently used for negative thoughts, activities, and behaviors, such as for emotional suffering, your brain will stop using those networks and they will fall by the wayside of unwanted past experiences like so much harvest chaff.

Your job, then, is to stop feeding the old circuitry that reinforces your fears and anger and, instead, direct your attention toward new, positive neural connections. Fortunately, you have the capacity to do that.

So, as we stated earlier—and it's worth repeating and reinforcing here; after all, that's how we build new neural pathways, isn't it?—becoming mentally engaged with an activity is requisite for learning that activity and strengthening the pathways that serve you in positive ways.

That is true in the physical world, and, as we will see later on, it's also the science that underlies your ability to connect with the divine energy field that permeates your existence.

But wait! The glass gets more full and the story gets even more exciting. Research now demonstrates that if you merely imagine yourself engaging in an activity, you can create the neural connections associated with learning it—without actually performing it.

In 1995, Dr. Pascual-Leone conducted experiments that compared changes in the brains of individuals who had practiced playing the piano, physically, with persons who had mentally envisioned their fingers moving across the keyboard. The brain changes in both groups were virtually identical.[7] The motor areas of the brain involved in playing the piano expanded in size in the group contemplating the activity, just as it did in those who actually performed the exercise. These subjects, therefore, demonstrated that the mere act of thinking about an activity imparted physical changes in the brain.

This means that you don't have to use old and well-worn neural networks of distrust, struggle, or victimization. Instead, you can direct your focused attention to creating functional neural networks for well-being, happiness, patience, trust, compassion, and all of the other positive emotions—but this requires a still mind which can be attained through meditation practice and the enlightenment techniques presented in this book.

You no longer have to live your life operating from the dark recesses of your limbic brain's flawed perception that the world is a hostile and foreboding place. Rather, you can establish new neural circuitry that will let you break free of a self-perceived destiny crafted by your family of origin, by early life trauma, and even by the states of health or disease that, according to the old, faulty medical paradigm, are preordained by your genes.

The discovery of neuroplasticity has become a focal point of unified interest in discourse among philosophers, scientists, and theologians alike. As Jeffrey Schwartz and Sharon Begley propose in their book, *The Mind and the Brain,* "The time has come for science to confront the serious implications of the fact that directed, willed mental activity can clearly and systematically alter brain function; that the exertion of willful effort generates *physical force* that has the power to change how the brain works and even its physical structure. The result is directed neuroplasticity."[8]

FILLING THE GLASS

This is where we explore the effect of mental attention *not* associated with any physical activity or dedicated to memory—that is, mental attention directed onto itself in such a way that we facilitate the experience of grace or enlightenment.

Andrew Newberg, M.D., director of the Center for Spirituality and the Mind at the University of Pennsylvania, uses sophisticated brain mapping and imaging techniques to examine how meditation changes both the structure and function of the brain. In his book *How God Changes Your Brain,* Newberg states that meditation not only modifies specific areas of the brain but helps the meditation practitioner behave and express emotions in a more positive manner.

Newberg's work shows that meditation enhances blood flow as well as function in an area of the brain called the anterior cingulate, an evolutionary newcomer that mediates empathy, social awareness, intuition, compassion, and the ability to regulate emotion. This structure sits in the front of the brain and wraps around the anterior of the corpus callosum, which is the thick network of neurons that bridges the two hemispheres. In addition to these functions, the anterior cingulate acts as communications conduit between the amygdala, which, as we've already stated, is one of the most primitive brain structures, and the prefrontal cortex.

The anterior cingulate thus stands at the crossroads. Its functionality, or lack thereof, helps determine whether our day-to-day behavior is reflexive and fear-motivated or is a manifestation of our uniquely human ability to recognize a wide array of choices, implications, and consequences. Newberg has quite graphically shown that meditation and other spiritual practices strengthen the anterior cingulate while also calming the primitive amygdala.

As might be expected, anger produces an effect quite the opposite from meditation. Anger shuts down communication to the prefrontal cortex. Emotion and fear determine and dominate behavior. As Newberg states, "Anger interrupts the functioning of your frontal lobes. Not only do you lose the ability to be rational, you lose the awareness that you're acting in an irrational way. When your frontal lobes shut down, it's impossible to listen to the other person, let alone feel empathy or compassion. . . . When you intensely and consistently focus on your spiritual values and goals, you increase the blood flow to your frontal lobes and anterior cingulate, which cause the activity in emotional centers of the brain to decrease."[9]

Bridging our primitive emotional response area, the amygdala, with our highly evolved contemplative prefrontal cortex allows the anterior cingulate to mediate how we perceive ourselves and our actions in relation to others and the rest of the world. Based on the fact that meditation enhances the functionality and capability of this circuitry, Dr. Newberg establishes a very important link between the physical brain and spirituality. He says, "We believe that there is a coevolution of spirituality and consciousness, engaging circuits that allow us to envision a benevolent, interconnecting relationship between the universe, God, and ourselves."[10]

Neuroplasticity is the link between contemplative practices and enlightenment. You train your brain to open the portal to wisdom when you turn your attention away from the everyday world and gaze within. In the past, it was thought that this ability belonged only to a few enlightened individuals, a belief system perpetuated by priests and religious hierarchies who had a vested worldly interest in protecting their privileged status.

In truth, every human being has the brain hardware needed to take this giant leap in consciousness. Our brains evolved to provide us with this equipment long ago. And if we look to the past, we can see the extraordinary feats of creativity and innovation that humankind has achieved by relying on the software that came preloaded in the prefrontal cortex.

■ ■ ■

Alberto:
Madre de Dios

Madre de Dios, the "Mother of God" River, fed by Andean meltwaters, lazily snakes its way to the Atlantic, 4,000 miles away to the east. The old man and I are lounging by the muddy bank, taking in the pink and orange sunset, the squawking of parrots a backdrop to our conversation. Our passion for the study of the brain has cemented our friendship, and our fascination with the human mind has brought us to the headwaters of this tributary in the great Amazon River system to meet the jungle shamans.

"It's baffling to me that nature compromised so much in the pursuit of consciousness," I say. "Think about how salamanders can grow back an entire leg after it has been cut off. It seems that nature has forsaken this ability in exchange for a brain that can become aware of itself." As I finish, I turn to look at the jungle shaman sitting next to me and see a smile come over his face. "And what makes you think that the brain created awareness?" the old man asks. "If anything, it is consciousness, or what we call *espíritu,* that creates the brain."

CHAPTER 8

NEUROGENESIS: GROWING NEW BRAIN CELLS

On top of the finding that we can create new neural pathways into adulthood, a virtual revolution in neuroscience has been launched by the recent discovery of the process of neurogenesis, the ability of the brain to actually grow new neurons. Stem cell therapy, a hot button of political debate and the focus of leading-edge research, holds the promise of offering a powerful tool in neurodegenerative conditions. We now understand that the human brain is constantly undergoing its own "stem cell therapy" through the process of neurogenesis. Every moment of our lives, several critically important areas of our brains are being replenished with stem cells that are destined to become fully functional brain cells, and there's a lot we can do to enhance this process.

NEUROGENESIS IN ANIMALS AND HUMANS

Because neurogenesis had been noted in various other animals, scientists in the 1990s were hard at it, trying to demonstrate that humans indeed retained the ability to grow new brain neurons. In 1998, the journal *Nature Medicine* published a report by Swedish neurologist Peter Eriksson titled "Neurogenesis in the Adult Human Hippocampus." Dr. Eriksson had finally succeeded in launching what was to become a revolutionary paradigm shift.

As Sharon Begley remarked in *Train Your Mind, Change Your Brain,* "The discovery [of neurogenesis in the adult human brain] overturned generations of conventional wisdom in neuroscience. The human brain is not limited to the neurons it is born with, or even the neurons that fill it after the explosion of brain development in early childhood. New neurons are born well into the eighth decade of life. They migrate to structures where they weave themselves into existing brain circuitry and perhaps form the basis of new circuitry."[1]

Dr. Eriksson discovered that within each of our brains there exists a population of neural stem cells that are continually replenished and can differentiate into brain neurons. Simply stated, we are all experiencing brain *stem cell therapy* every moment of our lives, a concept that remains iconoclastic in a number of scientific circles. His Holiness the Dalai Lama has stated, "It is a fundamental Buddhist principle that the human mind has tremendous potential for transformation. Science, on the other hand, has, until recently, held to the convention not only that the brain is the seat and source of the mind but also that the brain and its structures are formed during infancy and change little thereafter."[2]

The revelation that neurogenesis was occurring in humans and that we retain this ability throughout our lifetimes provided neuroscientists around the world with a fresh and exciting new reference point with implications spanning virtually the entire array of brain disorders. Alzheimer's disease, characterized by a progressive loss of brain neurons, had long eluded researchers seeking to develop ways to slow the inexorable decline in cognitive function that so devastates patients and families. But with the idea of actually regenerating brain neurons, a new level of excitement and hope was raised in scientists who were dedicated to studying this and other neurodegenerative disorders.

So, now that neurogenesis was proven to be ongoing in humans throughout our lifetimes, the question became clear: What influenced this activity? Moreover, what could be done to actually enhance this process? And the fundamentally important question: What can we do to grow new brain neurons?

■ ■ ■

David:
Journey into Neurogenesis

During my college years, I had the opportunity to explore the brain using technology that was just in its infancy. It was in the early 1970s when the Swiss began to develop microscopes that could be used by neurosurgeons to perform delicate brain procedures. While this technology was evolving and eager surgeons in the United States were anxious to adopt this new approach to brain surgery, a problem soon became evident. Although learning to actually use the operating microscope was relatively easy, the neurosurgeons soon found they were becoming somewhat lost when it came to understanding the anatomy of the brain from this new microscopic perspective.

I was 19 and just starting my junior year in college when I received a phone call from Albert Rhoton, chairman of the Department of Neurological Surgery at Shands Teaching Hospital in Gainesville, Florida. Dr. Rhoton was leading the way for the expansion of the use of the operating microscope in the United States and wanted to create the first anatomy text of the brain, as seen through the microscope, to better aid surgeons as they began to embrace this new technology. I had applied for the position of student researcher and was surprised and gratified when he invited me to spend the following summer studying and mapping the brain. It was from this research that we eventually published a series of research papers and book chapters that gave neurosurgeons the needed roadmap to more carefully operate on the brain. In addition to anatomy, we also had the opportunity to explore and develop other aspects of microneurosurgery, including developing innovative instruments and procedures. Spending so much time behind the microscope, I had become quite adept at manipulating and repairing extremely small blood vessels that, prior to the use of the microscope, would have been destroyed during brain operations, often with dire consequences.

Our lab had gained international recognition for its achievements in this new and exciting field and often attracted visiting professors from around the world. It was soon after a delegation of Spanish neurosurgeons had visited that I found myself accepting an invitation to continue my research at a prestigious hospital in Madrid, the Ramón y Cajal Center. Their microneurosurgery program was in its infancy, but their team was dedicated, and I felt honored to be assisting them in their groundwork efforts, especially in the work dealing with understanding the brain's blood supply.

The Spanish hospital was named to honor Nobel Laureate Santiago Ramón y Cajal (1852–1934), a great pioneer of neuroscience. Images of Dr. Ramón y Cajal were numerous in the hospital, and there was clearly a deep sense of pride among my Spanish colleagues that they could claim such an influential scientist as one of their own.

During my visit to Madrid, I felt compelled to learn more about Dr. Ramón y Cajal and came to deeply respect his explorations of human brain anatomy and function. One of his major tenets held that brain neurons were unique compared to other cells of the body, not only because of their function but also because they lacked the ability to regenerate. Thus, the liver, for example, perpetually regenerates itself by growing new liver cells, and there is similar regeneration of cells in virtually all other tissues including skin, blood, bone, intestines, and so on. But not so with neurons in the brain—or so stated Dr. Ramón y Cajal.

I admit that I was pretty well sold on his theory at the time, but I did wonder why it wouldn't make sense for the brain to retain the ability to regenerate itself, to have the ability grow new brain neurons. After all, researchers at the Massachusetts Institute of Technology had shown a decade before that neurogenesis, the growth of new brain neurons, occurred throughout the entire life-time in rats.

Soon after I concluded my research in Spain, I was off to medi-cal school at the University of Miami. And it was while learning histology, the microscopic study of tissues, that I realized how deeply entrenched in science was this notion that neurogenesis, while clearly defined in some animals, was not something that occurred in humans.

This teaching never sat well with me, especially when I thought back to my college years when the idea that "every beer you drink destroys 20,000 brain cells" was often kicked around late on a Friday night when surely more than that number had met their demise.

■ ■ ■

BRAIN-DERIVED NEUROTROPHIC FACTOR (BDNF)

A major component in this gift of neurogenesis—and it is a gift to be revered—is a protein called brain-derived neurotrophic factor (BDNF), which, as we read in previous chapters, plays a key role in creating new neurons. And it also protects existing neurons, helping to ensure their survivability while encouraging synapse formation—that is, the connection of one neuron to another—which is vital for thinking, learning, and higher levels of brain function. Studies have in fact demonstrated that BDNF levels are lower in Alzheimer's patients, which is no surprise, given our cur-rent understanding of how BDNF works.

But we gain an even greater appreciation for the health benefits of BDNF when we consider its association with other neurological conditions, including epilepsy, anorexia nervosa, depression, schizophrenia, and obsessive-compulsive disorder.

BDNF Activation

We now have a very firm understanding of the factors that influence our DNA to produce BDNF. Fortunately, these factors are by and large under our direct control. Increasing your production of BDNF and thus increasing neurogenesis while adding protection to your existing brain neurons doesn't require that you enroll in a research study to determine if some new laboratory-created compound will enhance BDNF production. The gene that turns on BDNF is activated by a variety of factors, including voluntary physical exercise—animals forced to exercise do not demonstrate this change—calorie reduction, intellectual stimulation, curcumin, and the omega-3 fat known as docosahexaenoic acid.

This is a powerful message because all of these factors are within our grasp; they represent choices we can make to turn on the gene for neurogenesis. So let's explore them individually.

Physical Exercise: Laboratory rats that exercise have been shown to produce far more BDNF than sedentary animals. But, interestingly, animals forced to exercise produce considerably less BDNF than those who voluntarily choose to spend time on the running wheel. Researchers have shown that there is a direct relationship between elevation of BDNF levels in the voluntarily exercising animals and their ability to learn.

With the understanding of the relationship of BDNF to exercise, researchers have examined the effect of physical exercise in humans, both apparently healthy individuals as well as persons at risk or already diagnosed with Alzheimer's. The findings have been fairly remarkable. In a recent paper, Nicola Lautenschlager of the University of Western Australia found that elderly individuals who engaged in regular physical exercise for a 24-week period demonstrated an astounding improvement of 1,800 percent in memory, language ability, attention, and other important cognitive functions, compared with an age-matched group not involved in the exercise program. The exercise group spent about 142 minutes exercising each week—about 20 minutes a day.[3]

In a similar study, Harvard researchers found a strong association between exercise and cognitive function in elderly women and concluded, "In this large, prospective study of older women, higher levels of long-term regular physical activity were strongly associated with higher levels of cognitive function and less cognitive decline. Specifically, the apparent cognitive benefits of greater physical activity were similar in extent to being about three years younger in age and were associated with a 20% lower risk of cognitive impairment."[4]

These and other studies clearly indicate that exercise enhances brain performance and is directly associated with increased production of BDNF. Simply by voluntarily engaging in regular physical exercise, even to a relatively moderate degree, you can actively take control of your mental destiny.

Calorie Reduction: Another factor that turns on the gene for BDNF production is calorie reduction. Extensive studies have clearly demonstrated that when animals are fed a diet with reduced calories, typically by around 30 percent, their brain production of BDNF soars, along with a dramatic enhancement in memory and other cognitive functions.

But it's one thing to read research studies involving rats in an experimental laboratory and quite another to make recommendations to human patients based on animal research. Fortunately, studies that show the powerful effect of reducing caloric intake on brain function in humans are now appearing in some of the most well-respected medical journals.

In a 2009 study, German researchers imposed a 30 percent calorie reduction on the diets of elderly individuals and compared their memory function with a group of a similar age who ate whatever they wanted. At the conclusion of the three-month study, those who ate without restriction experienced a small but clearly defined *decline* in memory function, while memory function in the group who consumed the calorie-reduced diet actually *increased* profoundly. In recognition of the obvious limitations of current pharmaceutical approaches to brain health, the authors concluded, "The present findings may help to develop new *prevention* and treatment strategies for maintaining cognitive health into old age."[5]

What a concept. Preventive medicine for the brain. While the tenets of preventive medicine have seemingly taken hold in so many other areas of health care, from heart disease to breast cancer, for some reason the brain has always been left out. Gratefully, with these new research findings, that is changing.

Further evidence supporting the role of calorie reduction to strengthen the brain and provide more resistance to degenerative disease comes from Mark P. Mattson at the National Institute on Aging Gerontology Research Center, who reports, "Epidemiological data suggest that individuals with a low calorie intake may have a reduced risk of stroke and neurodegenerative disorders. There is a strong correlation between per capita food consumption and risk for Alzheimer's disease and stroke. Data from population-based case control studies showed that individuals with the lowest daily calorie intakes had the lowest risk of Alzheimer's disease and Parkinson's disease. In a population-based longitudinal prospective study of Nigerian families in which some members moved to the United States, it was shown that the incidence of Alzheimer's disease among individuals living in the United States was increased compared to their relatives who remained in Nigeria."[6]

The Nigerians who moved to the United States were obviously genetically the same as their relatives who remained in Nigeria. Only their environment changed. And this research clearly focused on the detrimental effects on brain health as a consequence of the increase in calorie consumption.

While the prospect of reducing calorie intake by 30 percent may seem daunting, consider that Americans now consume an average of 523 more calories daily than in 1970. Current United Nations estimates show that the average American adult consumes 3,770 calories each day. In contrast, most health-care professionals consider normal calorie consumption (i.e., the amount of calories needed to maintain body weight) to be around 2,000 calories daily for women and 2,550 for men, obviously with higher or lower requirements depending on level of exercise. A 30 percent reduction of calories from an average of 3,770 per day provides 2,640 calories, still more than a normal minimum requirement.

Much of the calorie increase in Americans comes from our overwhelming increase in sugar consumption. The average American now eats and drinks an incredible 160 pounds of refined sugar each year, which represents a 25 percent increase in just the last three decades. This becomes particularly troubling in light of animal research done at UCLA showing a strong link between "the typical diet of most industrialized Western societies rich in saturated fat and refined sugar" and reduced BDNF levels and, as expected, correspondingly reduced memory function.

Lowering sugar intake alone might go a long way toward achieving a meaningful reduction in calorie consumption; weight loss would likely be a side benefit. Indeed, obesity, in and of itself, is associated with reduced levels of BDNF, as is elevated blood sugar, a common consequence of obesity. Furthermore, increasing BDNF provides the added benefit of actually reducing the appetite.

We hope that this data and the desire to help your brain turn on BDNF production will motivate you to follow a reduced-calorie diet. But, if you want to do more, you can implement a program of intermittent fasting, which we will describe in Chapter 14.

Intellectual Stimulation: BDNF is described as a neuronal trophic factor, which means that it is a chemical that induces positive growth, health, and functionality in the target tissue—in this case, brain neurons. So it would only make sense to expect BDNF to increase when the brain is challenged. Just as muscles will gain strength and thus functionality when exercised, the brain also rises to the challenges of intellectually stimulating circumstances by becoming faster and more efficient as well as having a greater capacity for information storage.

These positive features are all facilitated by the increase in BDNF caused by stimulating activities. Inversely, it is likely that BDNF levels are low in individuals who spend several hours each day watching television, playing rote computer games, or otherwise engaged in mindless and passive activities.

An agile mind is also a good deterrent to help us avoid debilitating diseases associated with old age. Mark Mattson suggests that agility education and linguistics are two ways to keep an active, functional mind. He states, "In regards to aging and age-related neurodegenerative disorders, the available data suggest that those behaviors that enhance dendritic complexity and synaptic plasticity also promote successful aging and decrease risk of neurodegenerative disorders. For example, there is an inverse relationship between educational level and risk for Alzheimer's disease; people with more education have a lower risk. Protection against Alzheimer's disease, and perhaps other age-related neurodegenerative disorders, likely begins during the first several decades of life, as is suggested by studies showing that individuals with the best linguistic abilities as young adults have a reduced risk for Alzheimer's disease. Data from animal studies suggest that increased activity in neural circuits that results from intellectual activity stimulates the expression of genes that play a role in its neuroprotective effects. Levels of several different neurotrophic factors, including BDNF, are increased in the brains of animals maintained in complex environments, compared to animals maintained under usual housing conditions."[7]

Being involved in stimulating mental activities—such as problem solving, exploring novel environments, and, perhaps most important, meditating regularly—enhances BDNF production and creates a brain that is not only more resistant to deterioration but one that enables you to push the limits of day-to-day functionality. In this context, it is important to view meditation not as a passive activity but as an active, brain-stimulating exercise. Even among Alzheimer's patients, the rate of disease progression is dramatically slowed in those who engage in spiritual practices, which, again, is likely a consequence of increased BDNF.[8]

Meditation helps us visit the complex environment of the inner mind as well as the universal energy field. And, not surprisingly, this might well be the most powerful stimulant for BDNF production. Meditation-induced production of BDNF should be looked upon as the fertile ground into which seeds of spirituality-induced enlightenment are planted and flourish.

Curcumin: Curcumin, the main active ingredient in the spice turmeric, is currently the subject of intense scientific inquiry, especially as it relates to the brain. But curcumin isn't new to the medical research. In fact, practitioners of traditional Chinese and Indian (Ayurvedic) medicine have used it for thousands of years. Curcumin is known to possess a variety of biochemical properties that include antioxidant, anti-inflammatory, antifungal, and anti-bacterial activities.

But it is curcumin's ability to increase BDNF that has attracted the interest of neuroscientists around the world. Interestingly, in evaluating villages in India, where turmeric is used in abundance in curried recipes, epidemiological studies have found that Alzheimer's disease is only about 25 percent as common as in the United States. There is little doubt that the positive effects of enhanced BDNF production on brain neurons is at least part of the reason why those consuming curcumin are so resistant to this brain disorder.

Curcumin activates the Nrf2 pathway, a recently discovered "genetic switch" that works by turning on the genes to produce a vast array of antioxidants that protect mitochondria. We will discuss this more in depth in the next chapter. This ultimately protects the source of divine feminine energy that permeates our physiology and fosters well-being. But credit for this knowledge is best given to the ancients who describe in the Vedic texts turmeric's key role in cultivating relationships with the feminine form of divinity.

In contrast, Western civilization is only now recognizing that the feminine life force, in the form of life-sustaining mitochondria, are the conduits through which the healing, nurturing, loving energies of the biosphere flow. Interestingly, only recently have we begun to suspect that these seemingly simple intracellular particles may actually be thought of as cellular manifestations of qualities that were once ascribed to the Greek goddess Aphrodite, the Hindu goddess Shakti, the Buddhist goddess Kuan Yin, and Christianity's Mother Mary. With this knowledge, we become intimately connected with our history and rekindle our respect for the gift of feminine energy.

Docosahexaenoic Acid (DHA): Perhaps no other brain nutrient is receiving as much attention lately as DHA. Scientists have been aggressively studying this critical brain fat for the past several decades for at least three reasons.

First, more than two-thirds of the dry weight of the human brain is fat, and one quarter of that fat is DHA. From a structural point of view, DHA is an important building block for the membranes that surround brain cells. These membranes include the areas where one brain cell connects to another, the synapses. This means that DHA is involved in the transmission of information from one neuron to the next and thus is fundamental for efficient brain function.

Second, DHA is one of nature's important regulators of inflammation. Inflammation is responsible for a large number of brain maladies, including Alzheimer's, Parkinson's, attention deficit hyperactivity disorder (ADHD), and multiple sclerosis. DHA naturally reduces the activity of the COX-2 enzyme, which turns on the production of damaging chemical mediators of inflammation. This inhibits the enzyme and helps put out the fire in our brains.

The third and perhaps most compelling reason for studying DHA is its role in modulating gene expression for the production of BDNF. Thus DHA helps orchestrate the production, synaptic connection, and viability of brain cells while enhancing functionality.

In a recently completed double-blind interventional trial called the Memory Improvement with DHA Study (MIDAS), some members of a group of 485 healthy individuals with an average age 70 and mild memory problems were given a supplement that contained DHA made from marine algae and some were given a placebo. After six months, not only did blood DHA levels double in the group who received the DHA but the effects on brain function, compared with those who received the placebo, were outstanding. The lead project researcher, Karin Yurko-Mauro, commented, "In our study, healthy people with memory complaints who took algal DHA capsules for six months had almost double the reduction in errors on a test that measures learning and memory performance versus those who took a placebo. . . . The benefit is roughly equivalent to having the learning and memory skills of someone three years younger."[9]

Humans are able to synthesize DHA from a common dietary omega-3 fat, alpha-linolenic acid. But so little DHA is produced by this chemical pathway that many researchers in human nutrition now consider DHA to be an *essential* fatty acid, meaning that health maintenance requires a *dietary* source of this key nutrient. Data also show that most Americans typically consume an average of only 60 to 80 milligrams of DHA daily, less than 25 percent of what researchers consider to be an adequate intake of 200 to 300 milligrams each day.

BDNF and Brain Protection

BDNF is important not only in neurogenesis and neuroplasticity but also in protecting delicate neurons from being damaged by a variety of insults, including trauma, transient reduction in blood supply, and, perhaps most important, environmental toxins. Indeed, in laboratory studies, rats and even primates with higher levels of BDNF are far more resistant to brain-damaging toxins than animals with low or normal levels.

One important neurotoxin often used in laboratory animal experiments, especially those designed to evaluate the protective effectiveness of BDNF, goes by the abbreviation MPTP (which stands for its chemical designation). This neurotoxin has the relatively unique ability to specifically damage a part of the brain in humans, as well as in several animals, that is associated with Parkinson's disease. Therefore, MPTP is often used to measure the possible benefits of pharmaceutical preparations to defend the brain against neurotoxins. But, unlike many other investigations that are developed in laboratories, the MPTP street story is far more intriguing.

In the early 1980s, seven individuals ingested a street drug they thought was similar to heroin. Instead, due to an error in the illicit production of the heroin-like drug, the substance they took was contaminated with MPTP. Shortly thereafter, they were diagnosed with Parkinson's.

While this was devastating to these people, it opened the door for researchers to develop a powerful experimental model for the disease as described by neurologist J. William Langston in his book, *The Case of the Frozen Addicts: Working at the Edge of the Mysteries of the Human Brain* (1997), which later became the subject of two NOVA productions by the Public Broadcasting Service (PBS).

Langston found that treating squirrel monkeys with MPTP caused almost immediate development of Parkinson's, with damage to the animals' brains occurring exactly in the same area as in humans with the disease. Subsequent experiments with other animals generated the same results. Langston and others ultimately concluded that MPTP destroyed neurons by destroying their specific source of energy production, the mitochondria. Thus, MPTP proved to be a mitochondrial toxin specific for the area of the brain associated with Parkinson's.

Once it was discovered that MPTP selectively damaged mitochondrial function and produced Parkinson's, researchers focused their efforts to learn how they could block the damaging effects of this neurotoxin and, presumably, by extension, reduce the damaging effects of pesticides in general. Various drugs were developed, including Deprenyl, that, at least in animals, held promise of providing some protection for mitochondrial function against toxins like MPTP.

While human trials showed only modest benefit, the most dramatic neuronal protection against MPTP was not found in some extrinsic laboratory-produced, patentable drug, but with BDNF, a substance already within our physiology, encoded in our own DNA, a gift not purveyed on a prescription pad but from nature.

Study after study has since confirmed that BDNF provides almost complete protection of brain cells not only from MPTP but from a variety of other mitochondrial neurotoxins. And in many of the reports, the methods by which BDNF is increased also come naturally: increased physical exercise and calorie reduction.

Thus, turning on BDNF production, through natural means and lifestyle decisions, provides our brains with powerful protection against the ubiquitous onslaught of mitochondrial toxins, such as commonly used pesticides, to which we are exposed on a daily basis. Obviously, choosing to eat organic foods is helpful, but we cannot totally eliminate our exposure to these dangerous and, yes, brain-damaging chemicals.

CHAPTER 9

THREE CONDITIONS YOU DON'T WANT TO HAVE

Oxidation, inflammation, and toxicity are not pretty-sounding words. Even if you don't know their exact meaning in relation to human physiology, you get the idea that they have something to do with producing a state of less than optimal health. Well, that's true; they are conditions that you don't want in your body—at least not to the level of being out of control and harmful.

Oxidation is basically the chemical combination of another substance with oxygen in a process that typically causes some pretty dramatic changes in the oxidized substance. As an example, rusting of iron left out in the elements is oxidation at work. And what happens when metal rusts? Essentially, it becomes damaged to the extent that it loses its integrity, speeding its deterioration.

Inflammation is one of the first responses of the immune system to infection or irritation. You've probably experienced this condition, too, perhaps as a sprained ankle. It looks like swelling and redness; it feels like heat and pain. Inflammation is your body's way of healing because, physiologically, it's caused by an increase in blood flow with an influx of white blood cells and other beneficial chemical substances rushing to the rescue of the inflamed area. Inflammation can also be associated with chronic arthritis, asthma, and neurodegenerative disorders such as Alzheimer's, Parkinson's, and multiple sclerosis. Medically, inflammation can be treated with topical creams and reduced through ingestion of nonsteroidal, anti-inflammatory medications (NSAIDs).

Toxicity is the state of being poisonous. Poisons, or toxins, are found in nature, including food, and in manufactured commodities such as household cleaners, solvents, and chemical compounds. We are even exposed to toxins produced within our own bodies. These endotoxins are dealt with by the multitude of detoxification systems that are concentrated in the liver but are found throughout the body as well.

Toxins, as you might expect, can cause disease when introduced into body tissue, yet, interestingly, organisms, including humans, produce toxins. In fact, some creatures depend on toxins for survival. Poisonous snakes, for example, use their venom to kill or immobilize prey, and some plants produce cyanide as a protection from being eaten. Because an organism, including you, produces toxins as products or by-products of ordinary metabolism, your body must break down or excrete them before they build up to a dangerous level.

Oxidation, inflammation, and toxicity—metaphorically speaking—also occur within society. Our thinking and memory can become "rusty" and we lose our ability to think originally. The angry, heated, pained old brain becomes emotionally inflamed; it festers and swells and generates rage. Potentially, the old brain's noxious beliefs and toxic emotional responses may cause it to strike out with violence that society finds unattractive, if not unacceptable.

Fortunately, there is a physical remedy for this metaphorical situation: antioxidants, inflammation reducers, and detoxifiers that help our bodies heal and facilitate our psyche's advancement from a state of primordial reactivity to evolutionary, and enlightened, reasoning.

ANTIOXIDANTS

Turn on the television, open a magazine, or listen to the radio, and you will no doubt be exposed to an advertisement extolling the virtues of some newly discovered exotic fruit juice that has the highest antioxidant content on the face of the earth. You may wonder: Why all the hype? What is the benefit of an antioxidant?

Antioxidants are any of various chemical substances, including beta-carotene, vitamin C, and vitamin E, that inhibits oxidation. In effect, antioxidants protect cells by neutralizing damage caused by reactive oxygen species (ROS), or free radicals. As mentioned before, free radicals are a by-product of the normal process of mitochondrial energy production. Under normal or healthy circumstances, antioxidants maintain a balance between the rate at which free radicals are produced and the rate at which they are eliminated.

However, free radicals cause oxidative damage to tissues, proteins, fat, and even nuclear DNA. In fact, tissue damage by free radicals is thought to underlie the process of aging. As we saw in Chapter 4, Denham Harman laid the groundwork for the antioxidant industry when he demonstrated that antioxidants "quench" free radicals in 1956. Then, in 1972, Harman recognized that mitochondria, which, ironically, are the actual source of free radicals, are also most at risk of damage from free radicals. Because the brain produces a prodigious amount of free radicals, it is their primary target, yet the brain lacks the level of antioxidant protection generated by other cells elsewhere in the body.

FREE RADICALS

Because of the powerfully damaging effects of free radicals, especially in regard to the brain, researchers are seeking better antioxidants that will provide brain cells with a measure of protection to stave off mitochondrial breakdown and, perhaps, enhance brain function as well. Studies are now appearing that clearly point an accusatory finger at free radicals for playing a pivotal role in brain aging. These studies show that, essentially, when a person begins to have too many "senior moments," clinicians apply a more scientific term, *mild cognitive impairment* (MCI). This phenomenon is generating considerable interest because MCI generally presages a more sinister pathology, Alzheimer's disease.

The relationship between MCI and free radicals was well described in a 2007 report by William Markesbery, a neurologist at the University of Kentucky, which demonstrated that cognitive function begins to decline well before the Alzheimer's stage and that the greater the oxidative damage to fat, protein, and even nuclear DNA, the greater the degree of mental impairment. Markesbery clearly identifies oxidative damage as a "therapeutic target to slow the progression or perhaps the onset of the disease."[1]

What a concept: to therapeutically target free radicals in an attempt to prevent Alzheimer's! What a refreshing approach published by the American Medical Association. Rather than simply describe some new drug therapy for a disease that's already well under way, here is a preventive medicine model, applied to brain health.

Markesbery goes on to state, "Better antioxidants and agents used in combination to upregulate defense mechanisms against oxidation will be required to neutralize the oxidative component of the pathogenesis of Alzheimer's disease. It is most likely that to optimize these neuroprotective agents, they will have to be used in the presymptomatic phase of the disease."[2] That last phrase means during the time of mild cognitive impairment or even *before* the appearance of symptoms. In other words, *you are never too young* to begin saving your mind for a healthier, longer "old age." And when we recognize that the risk of contracting Alzheimer's by living to be 85 years or longer is an astounding 50 percent, there are a lot of people who would be wise to consider that they are "presymptomatic" right now.

ORAL ANTIOXIDANTS

So, if in fact our brain tissue is being assaulted by free radicals, does it make sense to load up with antioxidants? To answer the question, let's go back to the mitochondria. In the normal process of producing energy, each mitochondrion produces hundreds, if not thousands, of free radical molecules each day. Multiple that by the ten million billion mitochondria in your brain and you come up with an unfathomable number—10 followed by 18 zeroes. So, you might ask: Just how effective is a vitamin E capsule or a tablet of vitamin C when confronted by this onslaught of free radicals? Are one or two little pills once or twice a day up to the task?

When confronted by a free radical, an antioxidant sacrifices itself to oxidation in a one-to-one reaction. Thus, one molecule of vitamin C becomes oxidized by one free radical. Yes, this neutralizes the free radical, but it also terminates the vitamin C molecule. Can you imagine how much vitamin C or other oral antioxidant you would need to take in order to neutralize the astronomical number of ROS molecules generated by the body on a daily basis?

As you might expect, human physiology has developed its own biochemistry to deal with the free radical fire. Far from being entirely dependent on antioxidants from externally derived food sources, your cells have their own innate ability to generate antioxidant enzymes upon demand when environmental signals to the cell tell the nuclear DNA to do so. Fortunately, this innate and internal antioxidant system is far more powerful than any nutritional supplement. Whether the juice of some exotic berry or an extract from a previously unknown jungle plant, antioxidant supplements are limited by stoichiometric chemistry. The golden key to antioxidant protection lies in your nuclear DNA. Now let's learn how to activate the switch.

NRF2 PROTEIN

Nrf2 Protein and Antioxidants

When the body experiences high oxidative stress and produces an excess number of free radicals, it also activates a specific protein in the nucleus called Nrf2. This is a very important protein, because it opens the door for production of a vast array of your body's most important antioxidants as well as detoxification enzymes. But what activates Nrf2?

This is where the story gets really exciting because the answer is: a variety of modifiable factors.

Vanderbilt University's Dr. Ling Gao has found that oxidation of the omega-3 fats eicosapentaenoic acid (EPA) and docosahexaenoic acid (DHA) activates the Nrf2 pathway in dramatic fashion. For years, researchers have noted decreased levels of free radical damage in individuals who consumed fish oils, the source of EPA and DHA, but this new research clarifies the relationship between fish oil and antioxidant protection. As Dr. Gao reported, "Our data support the hypothesis that the formation of . . . compounds generated from oxidation of EPA and DHA in vivo can reach concentrations high enough to induce Nrf2-based antioxidant and . . . detoxification defense systems."[3]

Calorie reduction, as demonstrated in a variety of laboratory models, also induces Nrf2 activation. When calories are reduced in the diets of laboratory animals, not only do they live longer, likely as a result of increased antioxidant protection, but they become remarkably resistant to a variety of forms of cancer. This attribute of Nrf2 further supports the fasting program that you will learn about in Chapter 14, "The Power Up Your Brain Program."

Over the past several years, Nrf2 chemistry has become a global focal point for medical research. This has led to the discovery that a variety of natural compounds activates and amplifies the genes responsible for the production of a vast complex of protective and life-sustaining detoxification enzymes and antioxidants. Among these are curcumin, which comes from turmeric; green tea extract; resveratrol; sulphoraphane, derived from broccoli; and the omega-3 fat, DHA. In activating the Nrf2 pathway, these natural substances enhance the body's production of glutathione, what may be the most important brain antioxidant in human physiology.

So powerful is the antioxidant protection offered by Nrf2-induced glutathione that it was able to prevent amyotrophic lateral sclerosis (ALS, or Lou Gehrig's disease) in the laboratory animal model of this disease.[4]

Nrf2 Protein and Inflammation

In addition to its antioxidant functionality, activation of the Nrf2 pathway turns on the genes that produce a vast array of protective chemicals in two other critically important areas: inflammation reduction and detoxification, which are also subjects of this chapter.

At first blush, the subject of inflammation might seem out of place in a discussion regarding enhanced brain health and functionality. But, while we are all familiar with inflammation as it relates to such disease states as arthritis and asthma, the past decade has produced an extensive body of research that connects inflammation with a variety of neurodegenerative conditions. Indeed, research clearly demonstrates a remarkable reduction in incidence of both Parkinson's and Alzheimer's in individuals who have taken NSAIDs for a number of years.[5]

Other studies also show dramatic elevation of cytokines, which are the cellular mediators of inflammation, in the brains of individuals with these and other degenerative brain disorders.

New technology now allows MRI and PET scan imaging of cells that actively produce inflammatory cytokines in the brains of Alzheimer's patients.[6]

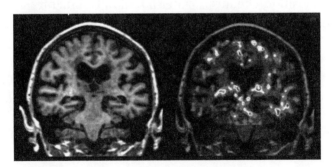

With this knowledge, we are now forced to regard inflammation in a whole new light. Far more than just the cause of your painful knee or sprained ankle, inflammation underpins the very process of brain degeneration. Ultimately, the key downstream effect of inflammation in the brain is that it is responsible for the damage that prevents activation of Nrf2 chemical pathways and the consequential increase of free radical production. On the positive side, turning on the Nrf2 pathway not only reduces free radicals directly but, as a bonus, reduces inflammation, which in turn protects the brain from excess free radicals as a result of inflammation. Do you see a positive cycle here?

Interventions designed to reduce inflammation through the use of natural substances, such as turmeric, have been described in medical literature for more than 2,000 years. But only in the past decade have we begun to understand the intricate and eloquent biochemistry that explains what traditional health-care practitioners have known and utilized for millennia. Indeed, food choices have controlled humanity's DNA expression for as long as our species has walked the planet.

Nrf2 Protein and Detoxification

The third and no less important benefit of the Nrf2 pathway is that it activates specific genes that produce enzymes and other chemicals that break down and eliminate toxins. You might wonder why your DNA would contain codes for the production of detoxification chemicals. After all, didn't humanity's first real exposure to toxins begin late in the history of humanity, with the industrial era? Well, no.

Some of the most dangerous toxins, such as lead, arsenic, and aluminum, exist *naturally* in the environment. Plants and animals also generate powerful toxins as a form of protection. Our human bodies also produce toxins during metabolism; even the carbon dioxide that we exhale is a poison to our systems, but, fortunately, it is essential for plants, which convert it, through photosynthesis, back into oxygen that we can breathe.

For these reasons, our detoxification system has served us for a very long time. Likewise, today, we are just beginning to understand how natural substances, such as turmeric, have also served as detoxification agents through their ability to enhance genetic expression. In fact, turmeric's ability to activate detoxification genes explains why it's also able to completely eliminate the damaging effects of radiation chemotherapies in laboratory animals.[7]

The human body produces an impressive array of enzymes that detoxify poisons to which we are exposed both externally and internally. Our DNA produces these detoxification enzymes, which have evolved over hundreds of thousands of years in response to our intrinsic requirements and as protection mechanisms for our ancestors as they migrated to new surroundings. For millennia, these internal defense mechanisms evolved, for the most part, somewhat slowly. However, over the past century, human physiology has been challenged by an incomprehensible array of novel chemical toxins for which our genetic detoxification endowment was unprepared.

It is as if we are functioning with outdated machinery, hoping against all odds that, somehow, our physiology will be able to deal with an unprecedented onslaught of toxins. And we are asking a lot of our body. But the good news is that we are endowed with a detoxification system with far-reaching potential. This is an important consideration because so many of the toxins to which we are exposed every single day are directly toxic to the brain.

GLUTATHIONE AND DETOXIFICATION

A significant player in detoxification chemistry is glutathione. It binds to various toxins and renders them less noxious. Most important, glutathione is a substrate for the enzyme glutathione S-transferase, which helps transform a multitude of toxins into forms that are more water soluble and thus more easily excreted.

Deficiencies in the function of this enzyme are linked to medical problems that include melanoma, diabetes, asthma, breast cancer, Alzheimer's, glaucoma, lung cancer, Lou Gehrig's disease, Parkinson's, and migraine headaches, to name a few. These deficiencies are inherited as subtle variations of DNA called single nucleotide polymorphisms (SNPs, pronounced "snips"). Various laboratories now offer a simple blood test to determine an individual's SNPs status for glutathione S-transferase and for other gene variations that may indicate an increased risk to disease.

Thirty years ago, Thomas L. Perry published a postmortem analysis of the brains of Parkinson's patients that demonstrated a significant reduction of glutathione.[8] Multiple other studies have since confirmed this deficiency, which further lends support to the idea that brain degeneration is a consequence of impaired anti-oxidant function. More recent studies show a strong relationship between Parkinson's and pesticide exposure, a situation that is exacerbated among individuals who are genetically disadvantaged due to reduced brain glutathione activity.

With this understanding of the roles of glutathione in detoxi-fication and as a very powerful antioxidant, as we will explore in the next chapter, it makes sense to do everything possible to maintain and even enhance glutathione levels.

■ ■ ■

David:
Outdated Machinery

When I was 16 years old, I became concerned about the mismatch between our inherited genetic endowment and the toxic environment that so characterizes our modern world, and I wrote the following letter, which *The Miami News* published 40 years ago:

"After spending three days and two nights at the Sebring car races, I found myself to be in question: Can we adapt ourselves to this future environment? Perhaps our bodies are more suited to the lush forest bed or soft sandy beaches where former humans lived in duration. I don't believe that the two weeks in the mountains or a Saturday at the beach will be enough to keep this body, which has evolved under less strenuous conditions, content. Perhaps the human will change rapidly in the next centuries to adapt himself to beer cans, concrete, and shattering noise. Our generations are each contributing to pollution-resistant lungs. But what about the people of today who are stuck with the outdated machinery?"

When I look at my writing since, I see that I am still challenged by this idea of helping people not be stuck with "outdated machinery." Take, for example, this short passage from the *Townsend Letter for Doctors & Patients* titled "Parkinson's Disease—New Perspectives," in which I expressed my concern for Parkinsonians whose physical machinery was not able to process and excrete environmental toxins: ". . . individuals with specific genetic defects causing hepatic detoxification enzyme dysfunction may develop Parkinson's disease as a result of exposure to certain environmental xenobiotic chemicals proving neurotoxic."[9] Fortunately, we now have the tools to override our genetic inadequacies and powerfully enhance our ability to deal with the many toxins to which we are exposed.

CHAPTER 10

CUTTING-EDGE THERAPIES FOR ENHANCED ENERGY PRODUCTION

It is the unfortunate activation of the process of apoptosis, or cell suicide, due to faulty mitochondrial function that ultimately leads to the loss of brain neurons in such common diseases as Alzheimer's and Parkinson's. Ultimately, these and every other "neurodegenerative disease" are really just variations on a theme. All of these conditions are manifestations of deficiencies of mitochondrial function, which leads to increased free radical production, which in turn activates the process of apoptosis. This is why so many leading-edge neuroscience institutions are so involved in studying how to protect and even enhance the function of mitochondria. Studies evaluating the clinical effectiveness of various interventions like turmeric and DHA, which enhance mitochondrial function, are now appearing regularly in mainstream medical journals.

Because mitochondria are involved in energy production, the science of enhancing the life-supporting energy production of mitochondria has been termed bioenergetic therapeutics. It's certainly a pleasant paradox that, after so many years, the seemingly infinite chasm between mainstream and so-called alternative medicine is at least partially bridged by the unifying concept that both recognize the fundamental role of energy in the equation of health and longevity.

HYPERBARIC OXYGEN: A KEY TO MITOCHONDRIAL FUNCTION

In Chapter 4 we described the chemical process through which mitochondria extract energy from food sources and store it in adenosine triphosphate (ATP). Oxygen is a key component in this function that powers each cell, every tissue, every organ, and every system in your body.

Because of oxygen's life-sustaining role for cells and indeed all life, scientists began to explore the use of oxygen as a therapeutic tool in the late 1700s. In 1798, Thomas Beddoes, an English physician, founded the Pneumatic Institution, where inhaled oxygen was offered as a treatment for a variety of diseases. But not until 150 years later did researchers realize that the real gift of oxygen therapy occurs when it is administered in a closed environment in which the pressure can be increased.

Administering oxygen in this fashion is called hyperbaric oxygen, and it first found its way into clinical medicine in 1956 when hyperbaric oxygen therapy (HBOT) began to be used quite effectively after heart surgery. Soon thereafter, the Western medical community explored the application of HBOT in a wide variety of clinical areas. They extolled the virtues of this new therapy, stating that it worked, fundamentally, by enhancing mitochondrial function.

Organizations formed to help clinicians study the new technology and share experiences. Divers benefitted substantially from HBOT because it alleviates injuries caused by a buildup of nitrogen in the blood after ascending from deep water too quickly. Soon, clinicians founded the Undersea and Hyperbaric Medical Society, which, in 1967, developed HBOT protocols for the treatment of numerous diseases from radiation injury to infected bones to diabetic skin ulcers.

But it has only been in the last decade that the depth of the potential for HBOT in enhancing brain function has started to become apparent. With the understanding that brain function is so highly dependent upon optimal mitochondrial function, the idea of implementing HBOT in protocols has been seized upon by many forward-looking neuroscientists. Delivering life-sustaining and energy-producing oxygen under pressure has been described as "potentially the most powerful brain enhancing technology of the 21st century."[1] I recall the late Richard Neubauer, who pioneered the use of hyperbaric medicine in brain disorders, stating on many occasions that the future of neurology is hyperbaric medicine, and the future of hyperbaric medicine is neurology.

Clearly, Dr. Neubauer was prescient. Studies from around the globe demonstrate that indeed the brain responds favorably to HBOT: benefits are now documented for patients with Parkinson's, stroke, cerebral palsy, multiple sclerosis, carbon monoxide poisoning, traumatic brain injuries, and many more brain disorders.

HBOT is on the leading edge of 21st-century medical technology. And, yet, it provides the perfect complement to ancient spiritual practices developed by shamans centuries ago. To emphasize again, hyperbaric oxygen therapy empowers mitochondria to energize the brain. It is as if a light switch inside the brain is suddenly flipped to the on position. This is why we employ HBOT, along with specific neuronutrients and fasting, as an integral part of our intensive prevention and recovery programs—with great success.

When mitochondrial function is enhanced, the brain immediately transforms itself into a far more perceptive system, opening the door for you to benefit from a far deeper experience when you immerse yourself in spiritual practices.

■ ■ ■

Alberto:
20 Feet Under

When I was young, I used to go diving frequently. Having been born and raised on a Caribbean island (Cuba), I was often in the ocean and felt as comfortable in the weightless underwater environment as I did on dry land. So when David first invited me to try out the HBOT chamber, I was certain I would feel at ease in the pressurized environment. I knew that under 1.5 atmospheres of pressure (equivalent to being 17 feet under water) cells receive as much as 20 times more oxygen than is normally available to them. This is because the normal oxygen transport system in the blood, hemoglobin, is easily saturated. But under 1.5 atmospheres, blood plasma becomes an oxygen transporter.

David's invitation came at a perfect time because I had been under a tremendous amount of stress. In the last seven weeks, I had been lecturing in Australia, Germany, and several U.S. cities. My body wasn't sure anymore whether it wanted to eat or sleep, and I could literally use a "breath of fresh air."

The HBOT chamber is an acrylic plastic tube with a narrow bed inside. As the nurse helped me onto the gurney and pushed me into the chamber, the thought crossed my mind that I was entering a fishbowl. Soon, with a whoosh, oxygen filled the chamber, and along with it came the familiar feeling of descending into the depths. Yet unlike scuba diving, where you breathe compressed air, I would be breathing 100 percent oxygen for the next hour. I focused on taking deep, rhythmic breaths, even though my system demanded very little oxygen because I was at rest. I wanted to make sure to get as much oxygen into every one of my brain cells as I could!

While David had a thriving practice and an international reputation for his work with patients suffering from degenerative brain disorders, I was interested in exploring optimal brain function. I knew that David had a strong interest in prevention and that a number of his patients with Alzheimer's or Parkinson's in their families actually came once or twice yearly for HBOT as a preventive measure.

After a few minutes, I began to practice mental gymnastics. I have never been very good at math and tried to do some complex arithmetic, to no avail. Definitely the "math centers" in my brain were not getting any benefit from the enriched atmosphere. But after a few more minutes, I noticed that I was able to recall the telephone numbers my family had when I was six years old, as well as our street address, even though I had not thought of these facts in many years. Long-term memory recall seemed great. I could imagine neurons that had lain dormant for decades beginning to fire, awash in life-sustaining oxygen. Yet, long-term memory is not lost as a result of aging. What is lost most commonly is short-term recall.

I have a notoriously bad memory for names, but I never forget a face or the stories that people tell me. Yet, with all my recent traveling, I was having a difficult time sorting out whom I had met in which of the cities I had been in over the last few weeks. So I began to reconstruct my itinerary city by city, meeting by meeting, talk by talk, and I found that I recalled them effortlessly, picturing them in great detail that even included the smell of rain in London. This was beginning to get interesting.

I had to consciously focus on taking deep, regular breaths because my oxygen-saturated body hardly needed any of this stuff to perform its survival functions. Next, I wanted to test episodic memory recall. Episodic memory refers to recalling a time, a place, and the feelings experienced; it is, in a sense, like traveling back in time and reexperiencing events. I knew that it was easy to do this with emotionally charged memories, as I remembered many of my patients reminiscing about all the times when they wished they had done things differently in the past, as well as a few times I would like to have done things differently myself. While all of these emotionally charged memories were readily available to me, I chose to focus on my childhood. I could easily revisit events of my past and recall feelings of that moment—when my dog was hit by a car, or when I went swimming in the ocean at the age of five and my cousin cried, "Shark!" and I breathlessly got out of the water.

Yet, there was a period of my childhood, between the years of eight and ten, of which I had very little recall. Because I had lucid recall of most other times, I suspected that I must have suffered some kind of trauma for my mind to block out these years. I could feel my heart racing as I decided to try to pry open these gates of memory that lay locked in my subconscious.

I recalled my grandmother and imagined myself with her. My grandmother had always been a solid presence in our home, even during the tumultuous times of the Cuban Revolution, when there was fighting in the streets and a great deal of family blood-shed. Soon, to my surprise, I felt tears running down my cheek. I recalled the fear I had felt as a child, knowing that militiamen could come at any time and take my parents away. Yet, I was wit-nessing that time as a grown man, observing the frightened child sitting on his grandmother's lap. Both of us were there, and I spoke softly to the boy and told him that he would be okay, that nothing would happen to him or his loved ones.

At the end of my HBOT session, I mentioned to David how important it was for me to remain alert and *breathing deeply* in that oxygen-rich atmosphere, instead of watching a movie or going to sleep, as many other patients did, which would reduce the amount of oxygen intake into the system. And I decided that, for the next session, I would attempt even more complex tasks under the influ-ence of pure oxygen.

■ ■ ■

GLUTATHIONE: MANNA FOR MITOCHONDRIA

Here again we shout the praises of glutathione, which, in addition to playing a critical role in detoxification, has also been termed "the master antioxidant" in human physiology. It is so important that scientists often measure cellular glutathione levels as an overall indicator of cellular health. And nowhere is its power more important than in the protection of the brain. While the brain represents only 2 percent of human body weight, it con-sumes up to 20 percent of its energy calories when at rest. This disproportionately high level of metabolism and production of free radical by-products puts the brain at great risk.

No tissue, including protein, DNA, and fat, is immune to risk from free radical damage, and fat is of special concern because it comprises 70 percent the human brain's dry weight and because it is one of the most difficult tissues to protect from free radical damage. Fat is actually a delicate chemical, and, when it is damaged by free radicals, it basically becomes rancid. In the brain, this translates into compromised function, which limits the ability of neurons to communicate with each other.

As we've mentioned before, free radical damage underlies all degenerative conditions of the brain, including Alzheimer's, Parkinson's, amyotrophic lateral sclerosis (ALS, or Lou Gehrig's disease), multiple sclerosis, and even generic brain aging.

In addition, the danger of free radicals is twofold. First, as mentioned, these reactive chemicals directly modify the various tissues that they attack, rendering them unable to function properly. Second, free radical action initiates apoptosis, through which the cell unlocks DNA-encoded instructions to commit suicide. So the antioxidant protection offered by glutathione deserves center stage.

Not only is glutathione a powerful antioxidant in its own right, but it also regenerates another important brain antioxidant: vitamin C, which recharges the brain's allotment of the powerful fat-soluble alpha-tocopherol, a member of the vitamin E family.

With its connections to so many other health-related chemicals and vitamins, glutathione is a prime focus for brain researchers around the world.

■ ■ ■

David:
My Introduction to Glutathione

"Fibromyalgia," the lecturer claimed, "is essentially a disorder of mitochondrial function. This explains why these patients are fatigued and why they are mentally fogged. Because the mitochondria aren't working up to speed, there is an accumulation of toxic by-products of metabolism in the soft tissues, and this explains the pain."

It was way back in 1997 when I attended this lecture offering an alternative medicine approach to what was becoming a fairly widespread medical condition.

Unfortunately for many patients suffering from this disease at that time, mainstream medicine flat-out denied its existence. When standard laboratory tests failed to show any evidence of abnormality, primary care doctors tended to conclude that the problem was "all in the head."

As is so often the case with "modern medicine," fibromyalgia became validated as a true medical condition only when pharmaceutical manufacturers developed a drug to treat it. These days, doctors simply write a prescription, and the drugs are flying off the shelves.

But the idea that problems with mitochondrial function play an important role in this disorder has maintained traction over the years, at least with more enlightened physicians who are concerned with treating the underlying causes of disease, rather than simply focusing on symptom management.

Shortly after the lecture, I returned to my office in Naples and began to reassess my approach to fibromyalgia. Coincidentally, at that time I was investigating a variety of techniques designed to enhance mitochondrial function and turned my attention to glutathione, a chemical normally produced in the body that protects mitochondria and maintains their function. My research revealed that glutathione could be administered intravenously and was approved as an emergency treatment for acetaminophen overdose. I was soon able to find a supplier and, before long, began to treat our ever-growing number of fibromyalgia patients with injections of glutathione, often with immediate and dramatic success.[2]

One September afternoon, I had the opportunity to evaluate a patient who, unfortunately, not only had fairly advanced fibromyalgia but Parkinson's disease as well. The latter had compromised his ability to walk to the extent that he was wheelchair-bound. We moved ahead with our newly discovered treatment for fibromyalgia and administered glutathione into his vein.

What happened next forever changed my practice of medicine. About 20 minutes after the injection, this patient got out of the wheelchair and began to walk around the office. I, along with my entire office staff, stared in amazement until we noticed tears flooding his wife's face, at which point we all started crying, too.

My mind was racing. What had happened? Then it came to me: it was already well known that Parkinson's is basically a mitochondrial disorder, so treating him with glutathione was actually targeting the root cause of the disease. As I would come to say in many lectures over the years since, "We treated the fire, not just the smoke."

Louis Pasteur once observed, "Chance favors the prepared mind," and I was, and remain, grateful for this chance event with this patient as my mind, deeply involved in the science of mitochondrial biochemistry, was "prepared" to connect these two seemingly disparate puzzle parts.

I soon uncovered research that demonstrated that, in addition to the fact that Parkinson's is a mitochondrial disorder, postmortem analysis had proven that the brains of Parkinsonians were actually deficient in glutathione! Furthermore, Italian researchers had, just one year earlier, demonstrated dramatic and long-lasting improvements in Parkinson's patients who received intravenous glutathione. The researchers reported, "All patients improved significantly after glutathione therapy, with a 42% decline in disability. . . . the therapeutic effect lasted 2–4 months. . . . Glutathione has symptomatic efficacy and possibly retards the progression of the disease." And yet, perhaps because it was not a patentable drug, no one had gotten the word out to the tens of thousands of neurologists who treat Parkinson's patients every day.[3]

After this original epiphany, I began to treat my Parkinson's patients aggressively with this new approach—with continued success. I incorporated compelling videotaped examples of Parkinson's patients before and after glutathione therapy into various lectures I was presenting to my colleagues around the country— primarily complementary-minded groups, who responded wonderfully, with acceptance.

Interestingly, several times over the years, mainstream neurologists accused me of hiring actors to stand in for actual patients in these glutathione videos. These challenges always brought to mind these wise words of the Belgian Nobel laureate in literature, Maurice Maeterlinck: "At every crossway on the road that leads to the future, each progressive spirit is opposed by a thousand men appointed to guard the past."

Over the ensuing years, the science surrounding glutathione exploded, and we began to incorporate this powerful natural substance into a large number of our protocols, from combating the common cold, to treating multiple sclerosis, to preventing nerve damage in cancer patients receiving chemotherapy. And, as of this writing, I have trained several thousand doctors in the United States in our simple protocols of glutathione administration.

■ ■ ■

GLUTATHIONE: MORE THAN AN ANTIOXIDANT

Glutathione, in addition to its critical antioxidant function, performs a wide variety of other life-supporting functions. Christopher Shaw, a neurobiologist at the University of British Columbia, stated in his anthology *Glutathione in the Nervous System*, "Many of these reactions are crucial to cell survival. . . . One hypothesis [that of radiotherapist Dr. John A. Holt] has even suggested that glutathione is responsible for the origin of life. While this latter view seems likely to reflect scientific hyperbole, it may be difficult to overestimate the central importance of this molecule in the biochemistry of living cells."[4] These functions include the synthesis, protection, and repair of DNA; the synthesis of protein; the transport of amino acids; the metabolism of toxins and carcinogens; immune enhancement; the activation of enzymes; and the elimination of damaging heavy metals.

So powerful are the implications of glutathione for brain health and function that it is not surprising that mitochondria, the source of cellular energy as well as free radicals, depend heavily on glutathione for their well-being. In fact, scientists measure the levels of glutathione within mitochondria as an indicator of their vitality.

But even though mitochondria depend upon glutathione, they lack the ability to manufacture this life-sustaining molecule and must therefore import it from the cells in which they reside. Many types of cells in the human body are able to produce glutathione, but most is produced in the liver and transported throughout the body, even into the brain across what has is known as the blood-brain barrier.

The blood-brain barrier is the brain's security checkpoint. It allows nutrients and other positive factors to pass into the sanctuary of the brain while preventing the entry of potentially damaging chemicals and infectious agents. Not unexpectedly, when liver-produced glutathione approaches the blood-brain barrier, it receives a warm welcome. New research now shows that a specific population of brain cells, called astrocytes—so named because of their starlike appearance—actually produce glutathione within the brain itself.

INCREASING GLUTATHIONE LEVELS

Unlike proteins, which are constructed from hundreds or even thousands of amino acid building blocks, glutathione, a manifestation of elegant simplicity, is made from just three—cysteine, glutamic acid, and glycine—which means that it is a tripeptide.

With the hope of enhancing the body's ability to make more glutathione, researchers have explored novel ways of supplying these amino acid glutathione precursors orally. Unfortunately, most have not succeeded because absorption from the gut is profoundly limited, and most of the glutathione breaks down in the stomach long before it has a chance to be absorbed.

However, one form of cysteine, N-acetylcysteine (NAC), as well as the antioxidant alpha-lipoic acid, does show promise. Both of these supplements are available without prescription at health-food stores.

Faced with the relative inadequacy of oral amino acid precursors, or even oral glutathione, to increase glutathione at the cellular level, scientists have explored other avenues to accomplish this task. In 2002, researchers at the Johns Hopkins Bloomberg School of Public Health, led by Shyam Biswal, discovered what they termed the "master regulator" of genes involved in detoxification, the Nrf2 system. They found that turning on this genetic factor greatly enhanced the body's production of antioxidants as well as anti-inflammatory and detoxifying chemicals. Glutathione was among the chemicals most profoundly enhanced by stimulation of the Nrf2 pathway. In his work, Dr. Biswal discovered a totally different approach for increasing glutathione. He found the golden key, the switch that turns on the gene's ability to make glutathione.

Moving further back in this cellular function, researchers also learned what regulates the Nrf2 pathway and identified the specific natural substances that activate it. Soon, they identified plant-based nutrients, called phytonutrients, that activate the Nrf2 pathway, which in turn generates glutathione production at the cellular level.

These phytonutrients include the spice turmeric (curcumin), green tea extract, pterostilbene, and sulforaphane, a chemical found in broccoli and one of the most potent activators. This finding explains the so-called broccoli effect, a stimulation of the Nrf2 pathway by eating broccoli, that helps protect the body when it is exposed to cancer-causing agents. Sulforaphane, a key ingredient in the product Nrf2 Activator, is one of the most widely studied activators of the Nrf2 pathway and can be taken orally as a nutritional supplement. Pterostilbene, found in blueberries, is one good reason why blueberries have long been touted as an important addition to the diet for their powerful antioxidant properties.

Pterostilbene is chemically related to the more familiar and popular supplement resveratrol. But in many key ways, pterostilbene is far more potent than resveratrol. Pterostilbene, like sulforaphane and turmeric, enhances the production of key antioxidants that are critical for protecting cells against the damaging effects of free radicals, most importantly glutathione. In addition, pterostilbene has demonstrated powerful anticancer activity in a variety of animal experimental models.

The activation of the Nrf2 pathway by phytonutrients is powerful and has important implications for human health. Studies show that the switches that control the various health-promoting genes that are targeted by this pathway may remain in the "on" position for as long as 24 hours after being stimulated by an appropriate phytonutrient.[5]

This means that specific phytonutrients that target the Nrf2 pathway are a powerful means through which you can personally direct the expression of life-sustaining genes in your body. And because these genes code for increasing glutathione, their activation helps preserve and protect your brain and even enhance its function.

■ ■ ■

Alberto:
Deep Dive Two

For my second HBOT session, I decided to take my brain for a test drive again inside the oxygen-rich atmosphere. I had just received an intravenous injection of two grams of glutathione. As I felt the pressure building inside the chamber, I reminded myself to breathe deeply. I knew that respiration is regulated by carbon dioxide concentrations in the blood and that, in the oxygen-rich environment of the chamber, my body would feel little need to inhale deeply. I wanted to get as much oxygen into my system as possible.

The task I had set for myself was to come up with the outline for a new book I was working on called *Courageous Dreaming*. I had committed myself to write this book over a glass of wine with the president of Hay House, and he had sent me a contract without either one of us knowing what I would be writing about. The only idea was the notion that shamans are able to dream their world into being as the result of the practice of courage. It's essential to have an outline before starting on a book, or else you discover what you are trying to say by editing and rewriting; it is similar to the wise idea of having an architectural plan for a house before you begin construction. While I had a *feeling* about what I wanted to say, I had no idea how to go about doing it. I had already tried out the trial-and-error approach to writing years before with a book called *Futuremind*, which a friend dubbed *Nevermind* because the project never seemed to end, and was never published.

About 25 minutes into my HBOT session, I began to feel a great sense of clarity, and I called forth my assignment. Within instants, I began to literally *see* the chapters of the book taking shape in front of me, all the while with my eyes closed. I could read the title of each chapter and scan its contents. Then I remembered the only other time in my life when I had a visual experience like this; it was in high school when a few friends and I smoked marijuana and I was able to *see* the notes of the music we were listening to in front of me. Yet this time I was in total and complete control, and there was only the perception of seeing the chapter headings before me, all of them appearing at once.

I recalled reading about how Mozart would compose an entire piano sonata at once, and how he complained when he could not write the notes quickly enough. In fact, every year of his adult life, Mozart composed more music than the Beatles did in their entire careers. I clearly knew I was no Mozart, yet all of these thoughts ran through my mind, even as I paged through the manuscript of the finished book and smiled to myself at the familiarity of the material.

Obviously, I had been giving a great deal of thought to what I would write about, and probably my mind was accessing information I had already organized in my subconscious. But part of me could not help wondering if I might not have been "stepping outside of ordinary time," as many shamans claim they are able to do, to find the completed book and bring it back from the future. Could I have been accessing some relativistic time-space where my destiny was available to me? And if so, might I also be able to do this to find a future healed state for myself, or perhaps even for my clients, one in which they lived long and disease-free lives?

I was tempted to tap on the plastic tube and ask the nurse to bring me pen and paper so I would not forget any of the details of the outline of the book. Yet, this was unnecessary because I could summon the *entire book* into my awareness at any time. And it was not simply written text. It was laced with feeling, texture, color, and fragrance, as all of my senses came forth when I witnessed the text. As we saw in Chapter 2, this is known as synesthesia, or the crossing over of the senses, and is commonly exhibited by individuals who are savants. The deep cleansing of free radical "sludge" provided by the glutathione, together with the abundant oxygen, must have allowed my brain to attain a level of synergy I had never known before.

As soon as I came out of the HBOT chamber, I outlined the entire book, just in case. Four months later, I handed the finished book to my publisher in a slightly better and more improved version of the manuscript than I had "seen" that day in the HBOT chamber.

Today, I take intravenous (IV) glutathione regularly, as I have single nucleotide polymorphisms, or SNPs, that indicate faulty production of an enzyme (superoxide dismutase, or SOD) that protects mitochondria, DNA, and proteins from free radical damage. But even more important than "seeing" the contents of a book, the IV glutathione relieved me of a tremendous amount of stress. My mind was no longer taxed or aggravated by activities that used to make me upset. If the waiter who served me in a restaurant seemed to be rude, it no longer spoiled my lunch; if the driver in front of me was behaving recklessly, I no longer let it upset me. I found that I was becoming less reactive to situations that, before, would have dulled my awareness and elicited an emotion-laden reaction.

■ ■ ■

David:
Glutathione's Extensive Role in Health

Glutathione's functions as an antioxidant, detoxification agent, and heavy-metal chelator as well as its ability to regenerate important vitamins like C and E have justified our intravenous protocols for its administration at the Perlmutter Health Center for more than a decade. Glutathione is like manna for mitochondria, enhancing their function while protecting them from the damaging by-products of energy production. And because so many diseases are characterized by mitochondrial failure, it's hard to know where to draw the line in terms of limiting the use of this natural substance. As mentioned above, I have trained thousands to administer glutathione intravenously. Many are members of the American College for Advancement in Medicine (ACAM), whose doctors are listed at www.acam.org and can be searched by zip code.

Intravenous glutathione leads to an immediate improvement in mitochondrial function, and the symptomatic benefits of turning on the mitochondria are often miraculous, not only in patients suffering from diseases but even in healthy individuals who utilize this therapy in conjunction with meditation practices.

Combining both oral supplementation, to enhance glutathione production, and glutathione administered intravenously by injection along with hyperbaric oxygen, provides an unparalleled level of therapeutic intervention designed to enhance the life energy-generating potential of mitochondria. In the first Power Up Your Brain Intensive, which we developed in 2008, participants engaged in a weeklong program of intensive shamanic energy meditation practices. In addition to these techniques, each of the participants received daily hyperbaric oxygen therapy along with injections of glutathione. We were not fully prepared for the results that we experienced.

■ ■ ■

GETTING OUT OF A DEPRESSIVE SPIRAL

"Byron," a successful entrepreneur and owner of a chain of food stores, came to our Power Up Your Brain Intensive because he felt exhausted. And no wonder: he had been managing to make it through each day on a dozen cups of coffee, with the help of amphetamines, and then knocking himself out at night with Valium and occasional recreational doses of oxycodone, which is derived from opium. In other words, Byron had his foot on the brake and the accelerator at the same time. His daily cocktail of uppers and downers temporarily kept him going at his grueling schedule but eventually sent his nervous system into a depressive spiral.

Like many people we have worked with, Byron was self-medicating with prescription and street drugs to try to correct an imbalance in his brain and make up for dysfunctional mitochondria that were not producing vital life energy.

The first thing we had to do was to help Byron detoxify his brain and nervous system. The drugs he was taking are all broken down in the liver, and glutathione is not only largely produced in the liver, but is also a major hepatic detoxifier. We knew we would have to get his liver to come back online so that it would be able to help the rest of his body eliminate the toxins.

Alberto and his staff began the energy medicine treatments, clearing the energy centers in the body and restoring coherence to Byron's energy system. He was receiving up to four sessions daily, including massage, acupuncture, and shamanic healing. (For a more detailed description of shamanic healing practices, see Alberto Villoldo's book *Shaman, Healer, Sage.*)

The initial focus of Alberto's staff was to help quiet Byron's HPA axis by utilizing shamanic energy medicine techniques, to ensure that he did not function in constant fight-or-flight mode. Byron's HPA axis was so compromised that he lived in a state of paralysis, which is the customary response when a person is unable to either fight or flee.

After the third day in the program, Byron reported that he was feeling weaker than ever and could hardly make it out of bed; he missed two of his morning sessions. Both of us, Alberto and David, recognized that he was detoxifying too rapidly, thus overwhelming his system. Because the body's own detoxification pathways and systems are already overloaded, reducing the toxic load on the brain and nervous system has to be done with support. We ordered a lymphatic massage, which would help cleanse his system, gave him fresh organic vegetable juice, and asked him to rest for the remainder of the day.

The following morning, he bounded into our offices to tell us that, for the first time in many years, he had been able to sleep without medication. He looked cheerful and rested, and the black cloud that had been hanging over him since we met him seemed to have lifted.

Now that Byron had gained some strength and his body was detoxifying naturally, Alberto and his staff could really get to the deeper energy medicine. Our intention was to clear the trauma from his energy field that had led him to abuse drugs.

We worked with Byron right after his HBOT sessions, when his energy was strong and expansive. After one of his sessions, he told us the story of his alcoholic and emotionally abusive father and how daily incidents of ill-treatment from the age of 10 to 12 had marked him. As we cleared this imprint from his field—which we do without engaging in the drama of the story, because that is not important in shamanic healing—he started to experience inner peace.

On the last day of the intensive, he told Alberto that he had discovered his life calling: that he had come here not merely to own food stores, but to feed people real, living food. With that, he left the Power Up Your Brain Intensive with a new sense of direction and meaning.

Three years later, Byron is free from any drug use. He reports that his mind is clear, the brain fog has lifted, and he is able to sleep without the aid of medication. Furthermore, he is using the contemplation practices described in Chapter 13, "Shamanic Exercises," to maintain and support his new, enlightened life. Professionally, he now owns a very popular restaurant that serves healthy, wholesome meals.

CHAPTER 11

THE SHAMAN'S GIFT

Shamans believe that the world seems real only because we perceive it as such and that everything we perceive is a reflection of an internal map that we ourselves, along with our culture, have constructed about the nature of reality. These maps are stored in what shamans know as the Light Body, and what scientists call neural networks in our brain. Shamans know that if they wish to change the outer world, they must begin by changing the inner maps, by healing the imprints of disease and trauma from the Light Body. They believe that the Light Body is the blueprint that creates health or disease. But how far does this metaphor of a blueprint go?

Biologists now recognize that only 5 percent of n-DNA codes for proteins to build the human body. The other 95 percent is considered "junk DNA" because it is noncoding. But what if this other 95 percent represents the "library shelf" of genetic possibilities that we are not currently selecting from? Could we cure illnesses and maintain health by modifying our gene expression? And what if we could do this by healing our Light Body?

When we heal our Light Body, we can access a knowledge that is available to all human beings. In doing so, we could interface with the biosphere in ways we've never imagined, to upgrade the quality of natural information available to us and install it in the hardware that's been in our brains all along.

THE GREAT PERFECTION

Bön is the ancient indigenous spiritual tradition of Tibet. The lineage of Bön teachers is said to have been founded by Tönpa Shenrab nearly 18,000 years ago, predating Buddhism by many thousands of years. Tönpa Shenrab was born into a royal family and, according to legend, left the comfort of the palace and traveled to Mount Kailash, where he meditated and attained enlightenment. Even today, followers of the Bön religion venture into nature to fast and pray so they can heal their Light Body and attain a greater understanding of the workings of the mind and of consciousness.

An essential teaching of Bön, known as Dzogchen (or the Great Perfection), suggests that once you heal your Light Body with specific practices, you are even able to survive physical death.

After the introduction of Buddhism to Tibet during the 7th century, the Bön traditions, which to this day remain shamanistic, lost favor among the royal families. In 1987, however, the Dalai Lama, who is a master of Dzogchen, recognized Bön as one of the five schools of Tibetan Buddhism and forbade discrimination against Bön practitioners.

Dzogchen practice cultivates a Light Body that is free from the imprints of trauma and disease. This is known as the natural, primordial state of an unconditioned mind. In this state, meditation comes easily and infuses everyday activities. You no longer need to retire to a primordial cave or monastery to attain inner peace and joy.

As your Light Body heals and your natural mind establishes itself, you will start to attain an inner peace and equanimity that will radiate all around you. As you become increasingly enlightened, your body will become more luminous. People will notice there is no longer a figurative dark cloud hanging over you or a literal dark mood about you. Instead, there is a new radiance to your being.

THE EARLIEST SHAMANIC TRADITIONS

Tibet is nestled in the formidable Himalayan mountain range and was largely protected from the marauding armies that besieged most of Asia over the centuries. Yet it is outside of Tibet, at the ceremonial burial sites at the caves of Shanidar, in the Kurdistan, Iraq, that we find the earliest evidence of a dawning shamanic awareness. Archeologist Ralph Solecki and his team from Columbia University uncovered an elaborate Neanderthal burial site there, which they dated to around 80,000 years B.C.E. The remains discovered seem to suggest that, contrary to the general perception of Neanderthals as primitive, brutish creatures, they actually constructed elaborate burials, indicating an awareness of an afterlife. It is also believed that shamans at this site cared for the sick and injured, nursing them with flower and herbal remedies. Pollen samples suggest they used medicinal plants, including yarrow, ragwort, grape hyacinth, and hollyhock.

Many skills that we take for granted today were once considered mystical and held the general population in awe. If you were able to count past 20 without using your fingers and toes or were able to divide or multiply, you were considered gifted. The earliest evidence of counting comes from a wolf leg bone dated to about 30,000 years ago found by anthropologist Karel Absolon in Czechoslovakia in 1937.[1] It was notched with 55 scratches, with deeper grooves for the 25th and 26th, perhaps marking the time between the bleeding cycles of a woman of the village. The shamans were not only healers and ceremonialists who tended to births and deaths, but also the earliest astronomers and mathematicians. The oldest evidence we have of a society that understood the value of pi (3.1416) comes from the Great Pyramid at Giza, constructed around 2500 B.C.E. The pyramid has a perimeter of 1,760 cubits and a height of 280 cubits, which gives us the ratio 1760:280, which is exactly equal to two times pi. This coincides with other historical markers of the awakening of the prefrontal cortex, including the discovery of the alphabet. The first written texts refer to the value of pi, which would not happen for another 600 years after the Great Pyramid was completed.

The prefrontal cortex allowed certain individuals to understand the nature of time and predict eclipses and equinoxes, which would also have been impressive displays of precognitive skills to the less enlightened. Early astronomers, such as the Dogon shamans, were members of religious societies who associated the heavenly bodies with gods or even identified them as gods. The Maya codices, which are written in hieroglyphic script, included detailed tables for calculating the phases of the moon and the progression of the equinoxes. So accurate were the ancient Mayan astronomers that they predicted that the sun's elliptical path through the Milky Way will align with the galactic equator on the winter solstice on December 21, 2012, an event that modern astronomers have confirmed happens only once every 26,000 years. (The Maya believed that this cosmic event would mean the transformation but not the destruction of the world.) Yet, while Western science turned its gaze almost exclusively to the outer world, studying the motions of the planets, the origin of the universe, and the evolution of the species, sages also turned their gaze inward and studied the nature of the mind and consciousness itself.

TIMELESS AWARENESS

Shamans discovered that once our Light Body was free of trauma, our awareness could be refined to identify both favorable and dangerous events in the future. Those who developed these dormant skills were able to guide hunters to where buffalo would be grazing the following day, forewarn their villagers about an approaching tsunami, and lead fishermen to their catch—which gave them an elevated status of sages among their peers. Skeptics have gone to great length to debunk these prophetic abilities, but ample evidence exists that they were real.

One of the most renowned examples of shamans foreseeing beneficial opportunities for their people occurred in the 1800s when the United States government displaced the Osage nation from its traditional hunting ground in Missouri. The holy men of the Osage led them to settle on land in Oklahoma that consisted primarily of rocky meadows and barren hills, habitat undesirable to European settlers. Yet the Osage sages assured their people that the earth would look after them for many generations if they were to settle there.

One of the factors that made the land particularly unappealing was a black sticky substance that oozed from between the rocks and poisoned springs. Only later was it discovered that the Osage had settled on one of the richest oil and gas deposits in North America. In his book *Oil Man: The Story of Frank Phillips and the Birth of Phillips Petroleum*, Michael Wallis tells the legend: "One visionary said that he saw, clear as the summer sky, the death of the old ways. He saw visions of more white men coming, and he could even picture their strange machines, snorting and bellowing as if they were iron buffaloes."

The visions of their sages made the Osage people of Osage County, Oklahoma, one of the wealthiest communities in America. As the experience of the Osage Nation proves, some of our finest discoveries come about when we trust our hunches and correctly read the signs that nature shows us. The shamanic practices (along with optimal brain function) contribute to the development of intuition, which in the case of the Osage, translated into great fortune.

THE LIGHT BODY

There are many ways to exchange information with the environment. Some of these ways require nothing more than eating an edible plant or drinking water from a spring, taking a deep breath of fresh air, or basking in the sunlight. We now understand that eating ripe fresh fruit provides fuel to tissues and cells as well as information about the local environment and that drinking from a pure stream quenches thirst and tells our bodies about the ecosystem.

This communication with the biosphere also happens when you metabolize the foods you eat. In the West, we may think of bread, for example, as merely a source of calories but, in actuality, that food brings certain information to your body as well. That stalk of wheat that was kneaded and baked into bread that you consume has a biological memory that was informed by the amount of rainfall it received, by how well it was nurtured, and even by the hands that harvested it.

Plant and animal foods are not only calories or fuel but they also communicate information to your genes. The new field of nutrigenomics examines how foods convey information about your environment to your cells. The early foundations for this new science came from the understanding that, while our genes have not changed much over the last 10,000 years, our diets have altered dramatically. Thus, different diets lead to different patterns of genetic expression, which result in different proteins being manufactured as well as changes in energy metabolism. For example, a form of light beer was the only fermented drink in the Americas prior to the European conquest, and alcohol in the form of whiskey was completely unknown. This explains why many indigenous peoples are deficient in the enzyme aldehyde dehydrogenase, which is responsible for metabolizing alcohol and which explains the very low tolerance for alcohol among Native American communities. Similarly, a large percentage of Europeans who lived where dairy farming was common developed the gene that enabled them to digest lactose, whereas many people from other parts of the world remain lactose intolerant.

Over the course of millennia, signals from the biosphere—from air, water, sunlight, and food—enabled species to adapt to relatively slow changes in the environment. Looking at ducks swimming in water, we can see why they have webbed feet. Observing giraffes eating leaves from tall trees explains why that species has long necks. But why do humans have such large brains?

Why would nature select for intelligence and consciousness when brute force, large muscles, speed, and sharp teeth do so well for so many species? Dinosaurs did not disappear because of their small brains. They were doing extremely well and showing no signs of ceding their dominant place in the land and air to any other species.

It is widely assumed that dinosaurs vanished because of an extraterrestrial catastrophe—a large meteorite striking planet Earth—that occurred at the end of the Cretaceous period 65 million years ago and wiped every large creature off the face of the earth. The mammals that survived did so because of their diminutive size, not because of their intelligence or greater brain-to-body-weight ratios. In fact, for the more than 100 million years that dinosaurs ruled, tiny mammals, most of them no larger than a mouse, lived side by side with the great reptiles. Mammals were not a superior form of life that came to replace the giants. They were simply the lucky beneficiaries of a devastating extraterrestrial event. With the disappearance of the dinosaurs, the small mammals took over the earth and became nature's preferred form of expression for intelligence.

Suggesting a nearly mystical interpretation of Darwinian selection, we believe that nature selected humans based on the precept of "survival of the wisest" and not only of the fiercest and fastest. Why else would nature burden humans with a brain so large that it only passes through the birth canal with immense difficulty? Why are human infants born helpless and unable to fend for themselves, while a newborn foal is able to run after its mother an hour after birth?

The information we process from the environment is, first and foremost, concerned with eating, feeding, and self-preservation. But it takes a very small amount of brain capacity to deal with this information. Perhaps our prefrontal cortex will allow us to decode and download an entirely new set of instructions from nature. The sages of old believed this was the case. They believed their practices allowed them to upload new biological instructions into their Light Body that would allow them to heal themselves and live long lives.

These new instructions upgraded the quality of their Light Body and helped them to heal from disease. The instructions also had to do with anticipating future biological evolution, with breaking free from ordinary, linear time, and with learning to maneuver in timelessness or infinity. It is these practices that allowed Amazon sages to discover the formula for curare without endless trial and error, and Osage seers to lead their people to a land of opportunity that seemed barren and lifeless to everyone else.

■ ■ ■

Alberto:
Claire's Light Body

"Claire" was a photographer and writer. When she went to her doctor for her annual checkup, her physician discovered a lump in her breast, deep underneath muscle tissue, and asked Claire to return the following week for a biopsy. Having gone through our training program in energy medicine at the Healing the Light Body School, Claire immediately called my office to schedule an appointment. Although I had no openings for several weeks, I made time to see her on a Saturday because I understood how important it was to intervene before she was diagnosed and possibly labeled a cancer patient.

We have numerous cancer cells that appear many times throughout the year in our bodies and that are almost always eliminated naturally by our immune system. If we happen to be diagnosed during one of these instances, we can become railroaded onto a cancer patient track. To emphasize, I do not suggest that you not go for medical checkups, but I want you also to remember that your body has a tremendous ability to heal itself naturally.

When I saw Claire, after a few minutes of listening to her story I entered that deep state of meditation in which I can track another person's Light Body. I noticed a dark, cloudy mass of energy above Claire's left breast that had begun to sink "roots" into her tissues. These dark masses always indicate some form of pathology, and I was naturally concerned about Claire.

We performed an illumination, which is the core healing process in shamanic energy medicine. After a few minutes, the mass of energy, which we call an "imprint" or "signature" left by an earlier life trauma, began to dissipate as I extracted it from her field. I noticed, during the time I was working on Light Body, that

Claire was sobbing softly and tears were running down her cheeks. At the end of the session, I asked Claire what she was experiencing. She told me she was recalling the numerous times when her older stepbrother had slipped into her bed when she was a child, held her down, and fondled her as she lay there frozen, unable to call for help. It's not unusual during an illumination for feelings and images of an earlier trauma to bubble to the surface. These traumas leave imprints in the Light Body that later translate into physical disease.

The following Tuesday when Claire went in for her biopsy, the physician examined the new ultrasound and discovered that the lump in her breast was gone. He was stunned and later explained that these things don't just simply disappear. Claire simply smiled and said, "Yes, they do." He asked Claire to come back for a follow-up exam the next day. She has had physical exams every six months for the last few years, and all of her tests show no foreign mass of any kind in her breast.

I tell my students at the Healing the Light Body School that there is a difference between a healing and a cure. Healing is the business of the shaman. Curing is the business of medicine and consists of treating disease. Healing addresses the *cause of disease*, which is generally a trauma and the toxic emotions that separate the person from his or her joy and health. These imprints are stored in the Light Body, which I believe is a luminous "mirror" for the neural networks in our brain. And while many investigators believe that the Light Body is simply an aura produced by electric activity in the brain and nervous system, shamans believe that the Light Body is what creates the body, the brain, and the nervous system. The Light Body informs and organizes the body in the same way that the energy fields of a magnet organize iron fillings on a piece of glass.

Healing happens when we clear the signatures left by trauma from the luminous matrix that envelops and informs all life.

CHAPTER 12

PRIMING YOUR BRAIN FOR ENLIGHTENMENT

While the important roles of diet and exercise are well accepted in relation to heart disease, for reasons that are not readily apparent these considerations are virtually ignored in relation to brain health. And yet, the scientific evidence confirming the importance of diet and exercise as lifestyle factors that can be modified to support brain health and function is both abundant and sound.

Maintaining and enhancing brain health are obviously important goals, but keep in mind that these same dietary and lifestyle activities are your keys to directly influence the expression of your genes. They allow you to redirect the course of your genetic destiny, preparing your brain to receive and incorporate the benefits of meditation.

EATING LESS FOR BETTER HEALTH

Perhaps the most important dietary consideration related to optimizing the brain, enhancing neurogenesis, and providing a fertile environment for the process of neuroplasticity, so necessary for building new neural networks, is calorie reduction. The biological benefits of both fasting and overall calorie reduction are explained by:

- Reduction in free radical production

- Enhancement of mitochondrial ability to generate adenosine triphosphate (ATP) energy

- Increase in the number of mitochondria through mitochondrial biogenesis

- Increase in the production of brain-derived neuro-trophic factor (BDNF)

- Reduction of apoptosis, or brain cell suicide

- Activation of the Nrf2 pathway, which leads to reduced brain inflammation, enhanced detoxifica-tion, and increased antioxidant protection

Clearly, fasting and calorie reduction have vast and profound implications for brain health. Just look at the list of benefits. It is so encompassing that it's hard to imagine that modern pharma-ceutical intervention could even begin to address these issues. Yet, the effectiveness of these simple dietary modifications for enhanc-ing brain function and paving the way for clarity of thought have been recognized for literally thousands of years.

We are just beginning to grasp the enormity of the brain's potential. How often have we heard the myth that humans only use 10 to 20 percent of their brains? Regardless of the exact percent-age, the point is that between our ears is a tremendous untapped resource that we are just now beginning to learn how to access from *both* a spiritual and a scientific perspective.

Let's explore how you can gain access to your brain's fullest potential.

YOUR BRAIN'S EVOLUTIONARY ADVANTAGE

One of the most important features distinguishing humans from all other mammals is the size of our brain in proportion to the rest of our body. While it is certainly true that other mammals have larger brains, scientists recognize that larger animals must have larger brains simply to control their larger bodies. An elephant, for example, has a brain that weighs 7,500 grams, far larger than our 1,400-gram brain. So making comparisons about "brain power" or intelligence just based on brain size is obviously futile. Again, it's the ratio of the brain size to total body size that attracts scientist's interest when considering the brain's functional capacity. An elephant's brain represents 1/550 of its body weight, while the human brain weighs 1/40 of the total body weight. So our brain represents about 2.5 percent of our total body weight as opposed to the large-brained elephant whose brain is just 0.18 percent of its total body weight.

But even more important than the fact that we are blessed with a lot of brain matter is the intriguing fact that, gram for gram, the human brain consumes a disproportionately huge amount of energy. While only representing 2.5 percent of our total body weight, the human brain consumes an incredible 22 percent of our body's energy expenditure when at rest. This represents about 350 percent more energy consumption in relation to body weight compared with other anthropoids like gorillas, orangutans, and chimpanzees.

So it takes a lot of dietary calories to keep the human brain functioning. Fortunately, the very fact that we've developed such a large and powerful brain has provided us with the skills and intelligence to maintain adequate sustenance during times of scarcity and to make provisions for needed food supplies in the future. Indeed, the ability to conceive of and plan for the future is highly dependent upon the evolution not only of brain size but other unique aspects of the human brain.

It is a colorful image to conceptualize early *Homo sapiens* migrating across an arid plain and competing for survival among animals with smaller brains yet bigger claws and greater speed. But our earliest ancestors had one other powerful advantage compared to even our closest primate relatives. The human brain has developed a unique biochemical pathway that proves hugely advantageous during times of food scarcity. Unlike other mammals, our brain is able to utilize an alternative source of calories during times of starvation. Typically, we supply our brain with glucose from our daily food consumption. We continue to supply our brains with a steady stream of glucose (blood sugar) between meals by breaking down glycogen, a storage form of glucose primarily found in the liver and muscles.

But relying on glycogen stores provides only short-term availability of glucose. As glycogen stores are depleted, our metabolism shifts and we are actually able to create new molecules of glucose, a process aptly termed gluconeogenesis. This process involves the construction of new glucose molecules from amino acids harvested from the breakdown of protein primarily found in muscle. While gluconeogenesis adds needed glucose to the system, it does so at the cost of muscle breakdown, something less than favorable for a starving hunter-gatherer.

But human physiology offers one more pathway to provide vital fuel to the demanding brain during times of scarcity. When food is unavailable, after about three days the liver begins to use body fat to create chemicals called ketones. One ketone in particular, beta hydroxybutyrate (beta-HBA), actually serves as a highly efficient fuel source for the brain, allowing humans to function cognitively for extended periods during food scarcity.

Our unique ability to power our brains using this alternative fuel source helps reduce our dependence on gluconeogenesis and therefore spares amino acids and the muscles they build and maintain. Reducing muscle breakdown provides obvious advantages for the hungry *Homo sapiens* in search of food. It is this unique ability to utilize beta-HBA as a brain fuel that sets us apart from our nearest animal relatives and has allowed humans to remain cognitively engaged and, therefore, more likely to survive the famines ever-present in our history.

This metabolic pathway, unique to *Homo sapiens*, may actually serve as an explanation for one of the most hotly debated questions in anthropology: what caused the disappearance of our Neanderthal relatives? Clearly, when it comes to brains, size does matter. Why then, with a brain some 20 percent larger than our own, did Neanderthals suddenly disappear in just a few thousand years between 40,000 and 30,000 years ago? The party line among scientists remains fixated on the notion that the demise of Neanderthals was a consequence of their hebetude, or mental lethargy. The neurobiologist William Calvin described Neanderthals in his book, *A Brain for All Seasons:* "Their way of life subjected them to more bone fractures; they seldom survived until forty years of age; and while making tools similar to [those of] overlapping species, there was little [of the] inventiveness that characterizes behaviorally modern *Homo sapiens.*"[1]

While it is convenient and almost dogmatic to accept that Neanderthals were "wiped out" by clever *Homo sapiens*, many scientists now believe that food scarcity may have played a more prominent role in their disappearance. Perhaps the simple fact that Neanderthals, lacking the biochemical pathway to utilize beta-HBA as a fuel source for brain metabolism, lacked the "mental endurance" to persevere. Relying on gluconeogenesis to power their brains would have led to more rapid breakdown of muscle tissue, ultimately compromising their ability to stalk prey or migrate to areas where plant food sources were more readily available. Their extinction may not have played out in direct combat with *Homo sapiens* but rather manifested as a consequence of a simple biochemical inadequacy.

Our ability to utilize beta-HBA as a brain fuel is far more important than simply a protective legacy of our hunter-gatherer heritage. George F. Cahill of Harvard Medical School stated, "Recent studies have shown that beta-hydroxybutyrate, the principal 'ketone' is not just a fuel, but a 'superfuel' more efficiently producing ATP energy than glucose. . . . It has also protected neuronal cells in tissue culture against exposure to toxins associated with Alzheimer's or Parkinson's."[2]

Indeed, well beyond serving as a brain superfuel, Dr. Cahill and other researchers have determined that beta-HBA has other profoundly positive effects on brain health and function.

Essentially, beta-HBA is thought to mediate many of the positive effects of calorie reduction and fasting on the brain, including improved antioxidant function, increased mitochondrial energy production with an increase in mitochondrial population, increased cellular survival, and increased levels of BDNF leading to enhanced growth of new brain cells (neurogenesis).

FASTING

Earlier, we explored the need to reduce caloric intake in order to increase BDNF as a means to stimulate the growth of new brain cells as well as to enhance the function of existing neurons. The idea of substantially reducing daily calorie intake will not appeal to many people despite the fact that it is a powerful approach to brain enhancement as well as overall health.

Interestingly, however, many people find the idea of intermittent fasting to be more appealing. Fasting is defined here as a complete abstinence from food for a defined period of time at regular intervals—our fasting program permits the drinking of water. Research demonstrates that many of the same health-providing and brain-enhancing genetic pathways activated by calorie reduction are similarly engaged by fasting—even for relatively short periods of time. Fasting actually speaks to your DNA, directing your genes to produce an astounding array of brain-enhancement factors.

Not only does fasting turn on the genetic machinery for the production of BDNF, but it also powers up the Nrf2 pathway, leading to enhanced detoxification, reduced inflammation, and increased production of brain-protective antioxidants. Fasting causes the brain to shift away from using glucose as a fuel to a metabolism that consumes ketones. When the brain metabolizes ketones for fuel, even the process of apoptosis is reduced, while mitochondrial genes turn their attention to mitochondrial replication. In this way, fasting shifts the brain's basic metabolism and specifically targets the DNA of mitochondria, thus enhancing energy production and paving the way for better brain function and clarity as well as a deeper connection with the divine feminine energy.

Given that beta-HBA enhances brain function, Alzheimer's researchers are evaluating ways to increase the delivery of the valuable ketone fat to the brain without fasting. In a recent report in the journal *Neurobiology of Aging*, researchers stated that administering simple fats called medium-chain triglycerides (MCTs) as part of MCT oil significantly raised levels of beta-HBA in as little as 90 minutes after consumption. More important, they observed markedly improved cognitive function in patients who received MCT oil in comparison with those who received a placebo.[3]

MCTs are unique among dietary fats because they do not require bile salts for digestion and absorption, and are readily absorbed from the gastrointestinal tract without having to undergo modification, as is the case with longer-chain fats. Most commercially available MCT oil is derived from coconut oil, which is nature's richest source of this important precursor to beta-HBA. Coconut oil contains about 66 percent MCTs. Health-food stores across the country carry high-quality organic, virgin coconut oil. The designation "virgin" is important as it means the oil hasn't been heated during its extraction process and this prevents damaging the oil and making it less healthful.

Coconut oil, with its rich content of MCTs, provides another approach to modify gene expression and enhance brain function by improving mitochondrial function and enhancing BDNF production. These mechanisms provide fertile ground in which the seeds of enlightenment can germinate. How fitting it is that in traditional Hindu worship the coconut is offered to the Lord as a symbol of divine consciousness.

Fasting is powerful medicine well beyond anything even remotely considered by modern pharmaceutical science. Indeed, the concept that dietary choices are healing is embodied in this famous quotation from the father of Western medicine, the ancient Greek physician Hippocrates: "Let food be your medicine and medicine be your food."

The Power Up Your Brain Program includes total food restriction for one complete day (24 hours) every four weeks. During this fast, you should drink adequate amounts of water in order to remain very well hydrated. *Fast only after consultation with, and approval from, your physician.* Ask also for his or her direction regarding whether or not to take medications during your fast.

In general, however, remember that the purpose of your fast is to eliminate calories. Therefore, supplementation during the fast should avoid powdered meal replacements, protein supplements, or any product that contains sugar. As described in the program below, you will increase your intake of DHA and continue with turmeric on the day of fasting.

While any day of the month would be fine for fasting, the Power Up Your Brain Program recommends that you fast on the 11th day after the full moon, which is the day considered auspicious for fasting in Ayurvedic texts. We believe there is a special advantage to fasting on the same day as the many other people who participate in the Power Up Your Brain Program. When you fast with others, whether they are physically present with you or halfway around the globe, you enter into intentional resonance with those persons. This will make it easier for you to attain brain synergy as you, along with others, collectively awaken the capabilities of the prefrontal cortex. Please check our website, www.PowerUpYourBrain.com, for recommended days of fasting according to Ayurvedic and shamanic calendars.

The Spiritual Side of Fasting

Gabriel Cousens, a physician who founded the Tree of Life Rejuvenation Center in Patagonia, Arizona, attests: "I often observe in fasting participants that concentration improves, creative thinking expands, depression lifts, insomnia stops, anxieties fade, the mind becomes more tranquil, and a natural joy begins to appear. It is my hypothesis that when the physical toxins are cleared from the brain cells, mind-brain function automatically and significantly improves, and spiritual capacities expand."[4]

The expansion of spiritual capacities to which Cousens refers can be the result of increasing the number of mitochondria and their function due to the shift in brain metabolism. This functionally enhanced and increased population of mitochondria provides the energy to fuel activity in the prefrontal cortex of the brain. As the renowned yoga master Paramahansa Yogananda eloquently put it, "Through fasting, let your mind depend on its own power. When that power manifests, the life force in the body becomes increasingly reinforced with the eternal energy continually flowing into the brain and spine from the cosmic energy around the body."[5]

Indeed, fasting during spiritual quests is an integral part of the human religious history. All major religions consider fasting as far more than a traditional ceremonial act but as a fundamental part of the spiritual practice, as evidenced in the Muslim fast of Ramadan and the Jewish fast of Yom Kippur. Yogis also practice austerity with their diets, and shamans fast during vision quests.

Thomas Ryan, a Roman Catholic priest who directs the Paulist Office for Ecumenical and Interfaith Relations of North America, summarized the sacred dimension of fasting when he stated, "Fasting as a religious act increases our sensitivity to that mystery always and everywhere present to us. It is an invitation to awareness, a call to compassion for the needy, a cry of distress, and a song of joy. It is a discipline of self-restraint, a ritual of purification, and a sanctuary for offerings of atonement. It is a wellspring for the spiritually dry, a compass for the spiritually lost, and inner nourishment for the spiritually hungry."[6]

PHYSICAL EXERCISE TO UNLOCK
YOUR BRAIN'S POTENTIAL

Like calorie reduction and fasting, physical exercise also turns on the genetic machinery to make BDNF.

Scientific research relating exercise as an enhancement for BDNF production dates only to the late 1990s when researchers attempted to identify the link between exercise and improved brain function in laboratory animals. They found that when BDNF was blocked, exercise alone had almost no effect on brain performance.

More recently, human studies have confirmed that aerobic exercise imparts a powerful advantage in terms of brain function. In a recent Australian study reported in the *Journal of the American Medical Association (JAMA)*, adults at risk for Alzheimer's who engaged in a modest physical activity program for six months—150 minutes of exercise weekly—demonstrated much greater brain functionality than a similar population that was not involved in the exercise program. The exercise group, even after 18 months, showed improvements in delayed recall of a word list, a memory function, contrasted with the sedentary group's decline on this evaluation. The active group also demonstrated dramatic advantages in verbal fluency and dementia scales. Interestingly, the authors of the study reported that exercise alone decreased the probability of dementia by 260 percent compared with the most commonly prescribed Alzheimer's drug in America.[7]

In another *JAMA* report, researchers again demonstrated a much higher level of cognitive function in older women who exercised compared with more sedentary individuals. The researchers concluded, "In this large, prospective study of older women, higher levels of long-term regular physical activity were strongly associated with higher levels of cognitive function and less cognitive decline."[8]

The same issue of *JAMA* also carried an article titled "Walking and Dementia in Physically Capable Elderly Men" that concluded physical activity improved brain protection in men as well.[9]

LIFESTYLE CHOICES

The dietary practices of fasting and calorie reduction, coupled with regular aerobic exercise, are powerful epigenetic factors that modify the expression of your DNA. Choosing to incorporate these lifestyle decisions into your personal plan for well-being means that you are directly influencing the activity of genes that code for improved antioxidant protection, detoxification, and reduced inflammation as well as the production of BDNF. These lifestyle choices have paved the way for enlightenment for thousands of years.

CHAPTER 13

SHAMANIC EXERCISES

In addition to the physical program of calorie reduction and exercise, the Power Up Your Brain Program includes eight exercises that will help you redefine your life and advance you along your path to enlightenment. These exercises are now part of the curriculum of the Healing the Light Body School. These are a blend of the shamanic and the scientific, with the shamanic being the base and science providing supporting evidence. Following are the eight exercises in the Power Up Your Brain Program.

1. Creating Sacred Space is a prayer that contains an invocation to the four directions, Mother Earth, and Father Sky; we recommend that you perform this exercise prior to and after all of the other exercises.

2. Quieting Your HPA Axis will help you relax the parts of your body and brain that produce damaging stress hormones.

3. Reselecting Your Genetic Destiny is a meditation through which you can alter the course of your life, beginning with the genes you acquired from your mother and father.

4. Sky Gazing is an ancient exercise that will calm your mind and turn on higher cortical functions.

5. Radical Forgiveness allows you to forgive yourself and others who, you may feel, hurt you in some way.

6. Drawing Life from Your Dreams involves two exercises: one will help you recall your dreams better, and the second will teach you how to dream lucidly and direct your dreams.

7. We Are Our Stories is an exercise in which you write your life story then change it to provide you with a more positive outlook on life.

8. The Shaman's Bath is a practice that cleanses your Luminous Energy Field. Once a week you soak in a hot bath of healing and energizing substances prior to going to bed.

These shamanic exercises are explained in depth here; the next chapter outlines the entire Power Up Your Brain Program, which incorporates the exercises into a structured practice also involving neuronutrients, fasting, and physical exercise.

CREATING SACRED SPACE

People in the West think of sacred spaces as designated holy places—churches or temples, or perhaps a beautiful spot in nature. But the shaman understands that he or she can create a sacred space anywhere and at any time by focusing attention and summoning the power of the four cardinal directions and Mother Earth and Father Sun.

In doing so, the sage is able to come into relationship with the four shamanic organizing principles of the world: South as the place of the serpent; West as the place of the jaguar; North as the place of the hummingbird; and East as the place of the eagle. The sages believe that these animal archetypes are more than symbols; they are primordial energies with qualities and powers of their own.

Each of these animals can be seen as representing one of the four fundamental forces of nature, described by physics as the forces of gravity, electromagnetism, and the strong and the weak nuclear force. Biologists also recognize that all of the poetry of life is written with an alphabet containing only four letters: the four letters, or base pairs, of DNA. The only difference between the shamanistic view and the physics view and the biological view is that the sages believed they could summon and interact with these forces of nature, effectively communing with the biosphere. For this reason, shamans always begin their meditations and ceremonies by creating sacred space. Even if you do not use the words in the prayer below, turn to each of the four directions and *feel* a connection to each of the animal archetypes. Help your educated, logical brain understand that these are ancient personifications of the forces of nature. As you give yourself permission to connect with the four cardinal directions and heaven and earth, imagine the luminous web that connects you with nature and all of life.

Sacred space is holy and safe. You might imagine it as a shimmering cupola above the room you are in. This is a palpable space where you can lower the defenses of your older brain, a place where you can rise above its predatory consciousness. You might notice that others feel the calm and beauty of this space, too, as it defuses conflict and makes conversation easy and significant.

Creating Sacred Space is an experiment in the power of intention that enables you to summon the healing faculties of nature and come into right relationship with all the forces of creation.

Exercise: Invocation to Create Sacred Space

The opening of sacred space consists of an invocation, calling on the four cardinal directions of South, West, North, and East, and on Mother Earth and Father Sky. An invocation such as this is used by shamans around the world to connect with the living energies of the biosphere. Use this invocation until your own prayer reveals itself to you.

When you have finished your opening invocation, be sure to close the sacred space, as suggested below. This is the one we teach our students at the Healing the Light Body School.

Opening the Sacred Space

Face South and say softly:
To the winds of the South, Great Serpent,
Teach us to shed the past the way you shed your skin,
To walk softly on the Earth.

Face West and say softly:
To the winds of the West, Mother Jaguar,
Teach us the way of peace, to live impeccably.
Show us the way beyond death.

Face North and say softly:
To the winds of the North, Hummingbird, Ancient Ones,
We honor you who have come before us
And you who will come after us, our children's children.

Face East and say softly:
To the winds of the East, Great Eagle,
Show us the mountains we only dare to dream of.
Teach us to fly wing to wing with the Great Spirit.

Touch the ground where you stand and say softly:
Mother Earth,
We've gathered for the healing of all of your children.
The Stone People, the Plant People,
The four-legged, the two-legged, the ones that crawl on the Earth,
The ones that fly and swim through the waters,
All our relations.

Reach to the heavens and say softly:
Father Sun, Grandmother Moon, to the Star Nations.
Great Spirit, you who are the unnameable One.
Thank you for allowing us to sing the Song of Life.

Closing the Sacred Space

Repeat the invocation for opening the sacred space in the same order—briefly addressing the South, West, North, East, then Mother Earth and Father Sky.

Thank the archetypes—Serpent, Jaguar, Hummingbird, and Eagle—for being with you and release their energies to the four corners of the earth.

QUIETING YOUR HPA AXIS

The body has two defense systems: one to detect and respond to perceived threats in the external environment, and the other to detect and respond to internal threats. The first is the fight-or-flight response. The second is the immune system.

As we discussed earlier, the fight-or-flight response works through the HPA axis. When there are no perceived external threats, the HPA axis is at rest and all the body's resources are dedicated to the renewal of its systems and the growth of new cells. When the body perceives an external threat, such as the sudden roar of a lion or the blare of an automobile horn, the HPA axis kicks in and signals the release of cortisol and adrenaline, which constrict blood vessels in the digestive tract and redirect blood flow away from the internal organs to the extremities, preparing us to fight or flee. These hormones also constrict blood vessels in the prefrontal cortex, where our logic and reasoning centers are located, and redirect blood to the old brain, where reflex, instinctive action originates. As a result, our thinking becomes muddled and we operate like a cornered animal.

This is an ancient survival mechanism that continues to serve us well. The problem is that the old brain does not differentiate between perceived danger and actual danger. In our modern Western world, while we are not faced with many roaring lions, we are, instead, caught in frustrating traffic jams and toxic emotional assaults at the office or at home. Television supplies a constant feed of violence, and we remain in a hypervigilant state, our amygdala keeping us in high alert. Day-to-day life in the 21st century keeps us awash in a torrent of stress hormones, the most damaging of which, at least from the brain's perspective, is cortisol. In chronically stressed patients as well as depressed individuals, both the hippocampus and the prefrontal cortex are physically shriveled and shrunken—they were experiencing much more rapid breakdown of the brain than the their nonstressed counterparts.

The shamanic practice of quieting your HPA axis is a form of shamanic meditation, and can be likened to a form of relaxation employed in a recent study to determine if meditation could slow down cellular aging. This study examined the length of telomeres, which are the protective end caps of chromosomes and a representative measure of cellular aging, in two groups of mothers. One group was experiencing high levels of stress due to coping with a chronically ill child, while the other women had healthy children and experienced only low or what might be considered normal levels of stress.[1]

The authors discovered that the mothers who had been caring for their chronically ill children had shorter telomeres, which is an indication that these women had a more advanced degree of cellular aging as well as having DNA at higher risk for damage. The stressed mothers were aging much more rapidly than the mothers whose lives were less emotionally challenging.

The stressed mothers also showed low levels of telomerase, which are enzymes that restore and repair the length of frayed telomeres. Low telomerase is indicative of decreased protection of DNA and is associated with all the stress-related diseases as well as with cardiovascular disease, diabetes, cancer, and obesity. The authors concluded, "We propose that some forms of meditation may have salutary effects on telomere length by reducing cognitive stress and stress arousal and increasing positive states of mind."

That, of course, is the physical or scientific part of this story. From a shamanic perspective, we know that the chakras or energy centers are part of our luminous anatomy.

In the same way that we have physical organs in the body, the chakras are the organs of the Light Body that surrounds the physical body. They are possibly created by electrical activity in nerve plexuses along the spine where many spinal nerves combine into large nerve clusters. The chakras roughly correspond to the location of the body's endocrine glands, which produce hormones.

There are five major plexuses along the spine. The shamans and mystics around the world who were able to sense the electrical activity of these plexuses identified them as the lower five chakras. The sixth is the legendary "third eye," located at the forehead, and is linked with the pituitary gland. The seventh is the "crown" chakra located at the top of the head and is associated with the pineal gland. Both of these glands reside deep inside the brain.

The following exercise will help you relax deeply and reset the fight-or-flight response that might have been triggered by stress or trauma. You accomplish this by "tuning" your chakra system.

Exercise: Quieting Your HPA Axis

Do this exercise in a bathtub while taking a Shaman's Bath, or in bed before going to sleep.

Lie back comfortably and close your eyes, breathing in through your nose and exhaling through your mouth.

Inhale for a slow count of four.

Exhale for a slow count of four, drawing out the breath and making a slight whooshing sound.

After a few minutes of this rhythmic breathing, place your left hand on the center of your chest, at the level of your heart. Try to find your heartbeat, and bring your attention to this master drummer that sets the rhythm for your entire body.

Notice how your heart rate quiets as you make your breaths softer and longer.

After a couple of minutes, bring your right hand to your second chakra, right below your belly button. Try to feel your heartbeat here as well, through your right hand, even though it is nowhere near your heart.

Realize that the second chakra is linked to the adrenal glands, which produce adrenaline and keep the fight-or-flight system turned to the on position. Imagine that your heartbeat is setting the tempo for your adrenals, helping them to slow down and relax. Tap the fingers of your right hand softly on your lower belly to bring your awareness to this area of your body.

Practice for ten minutes.

RESELECTING YOUR GENETIC DESTINY

Modern physics explains that interactions across time and space are possible. Shamans learned to put this into practice and employed imagery to program their genetic biocomputer, selecting genes from the gene pool for health and longevity.

So imagine that you could go back in time to the moment of your conception and select the biological traits that you wish you had inherited from your mother and your father. Perhaps you would choose your father's heart because there was no incidence of heart disease in his side of the family. Or you might select your mother's brain because there was no Alzheimer's in her branch of the family tree. You likely would want the trait of longevity from either of them.

The Austrian monk and botanist Gregor Mendel discovered in the mid-1880s that plants inherit specific biological information from each parent. His observations led him to differentiate between the *genotype*, which is the sum of all genetic diversity in a member of a particular species, and *phenotype*, which comprises the actual properties and traits that individual members of the species express. Even though Mendel's theories were met with disbelief and he died in obscurity, his stature was later vindicated, and his discoveries are still relevant today.

You received the entirety of your genetic makeup at the moment of your conception. You also received one half of each of your parents' genetic code. This means that, while you received 50 percent of each of your parents' hereditary information, *their* genotype, you also express only some of those select traits, *your* phenotype.

But that is only part of the story. While you may have inherited a predisposition for either heart health or disease, your beliefs, diet, and choice of lifestyle will influence your inherited risk factors. As the pharmaceutical industry knows, lifestyle modifications are often not enough, and seemingly healthy men and women can and do suffer heart attacks at a relatively young age.

So, what else can you do? You can look beyond your physical or genetic side to your spiritual side.

Ancient sages developed techniques that they believed allowed them to "journey back in time" to influence the effects of their ancestral heritage. The effectiveness of this exercise derived, at least in part, from their ability to influence the expression of their DNA. In other words, they used visualization techniques to modify genetic expression! When skilled practitioners journey back to the moment of conception to consciously select the traits they want to express, they look at other factors—beyond genotypes and phenotypes—that may have influenced their genetic makeup. The father may have consumed too much alcohol. The mother may have been afraid of getting pregnant. The environment may not have been infused with love, peace, and tranquility. Stress hormones easily cross the placental barrier and inform the child of every mood the mother is feeling.

But now, from your current wisdom perspective, you can go back and visit the moment of your conception. You can bring a meditative and sacred feeling to the moment of the comingling of your genes. So, during this exercise, you can forgive your parents for any transgressions you believe they committed toward you, any hurt you feel they might have imposed on you.

This is necessary for your journey into enlightenment because holding on to any residual anger or resentment toward your parents only perpetuates your role as a victim of their genetic signatures.

Exercise: The Moment of Your Conception

With your eyes closed, take a few deep, relaxing breaths. Count your breaths from one to ten, then back to one again, until you feel yourself entering a deep state of relaxation.

You will notice that, at first, your mind will wander. You may find yourself counting past ten or chasing a thought about what you forgot to do yesterday or whom you must call still today. Let all of these thoughts go by like clouds that appear, then disappear, in the sky.

Now imagine your timeline, the chronological series of events in your life, poised in front of you. Perhaps you imagine a golden thread or a string with many beads or moments of time. Perhaps you simply see a road that leads in one direction to the past and another direction forward into the future.

Begin traveling backward along your timeline, briefly revisiting events of the past few days. Then go farther into the past, to your childhood, and to your earliest memories as a toddler. See the images as though they are in a movie that you can fast-forward or reverse at will.

When you are no longer able to recall events or situations, use your imagination. Imagine yourself as a baby in your mother's arms. Imagine being inside her womb. Imagine the instant of your conception, when your mother's egg is surrounded by your father's numerous sperm, all trying to fertilize it.

Imagine yourself sitting inside that luminous egg. It is a peaceful bubble. Bring your stillness and grace into that space. Know that you are filling it with your peace and luminosity.

Now sense the egg selecting and inviting the finest sperm to fertilize it. Imagine that as it enters into the ovum, you witness the most extraordinary alchemy that is the conception of *you*. You see proteins cross-link with each other, making the matrix of the egg hard and impermeable to other sperm. The nuclei of the sperm and the egg dissolve, and the father's DNA and the mother's DNA fuse. The egg divides and forms two tiny, identical cells. They begin to replicate, doubling, quadrupling, and exponentially adding to their numbers at an extraordinary rate.

As you watch this amazing process, you hold steadfast to your intention of forming and shaping yourself into your desired being. You bathe these nascent cells with your great peace, your serenity, your light. You bless this holy union that is you regardless of what the "facts" of your conception may have been.

And there, then, as the growing, forming you, you forgive your parents. You see them as the holy, glorious, innocent beings they are. You bathe them with your love, knowing that all is well.

You sigh. And smile.

Then, you return along your timeline to the present, bringing with you—into the here and now—your feelings of peace and luminosity, your joy and exhilaration, that you experienced at that moment of your conception.

SKY GAZING

The practice of Sky Gazing is at the heart of spiritual practice in the Tibetan Dzogchen and other ancient shamanic traditions.

During this exercise you leave behind your mundane affairs and your seemingly all-important to-do lists, and enter the silent inner world where all healing takes place, where your body's natural rhythms—pulse, respiration, brain waves, and energy systems—synchronize with each other.

Exercise: Sky Gazing

Sit in a comfortable chair with your hands resting gently on your knees, eyes open, gazing straight ahead into the horizon, at the sky. Relax your jaw and allow your eyes to look with a soft gaze.

Take deep, gentle breaths. Relax your belly, keeping it soft.

As you follow your breathing, observe your feelings, thoughts, and moods. Simply witness everything that surfaces in your awareness as if it were a cloud in the sky that appears and disappears of its own accord. As you inhale, note how you are the observer. As you exhale, notice how easy it is to get lost in thought.

With time, you will start to realize that you are none of your feelings or your thoughts but that you are the Seer who observes all. Notice where your mind wanders off to, and then bring it back gently to focus on your breath as you gaze at the morning sky.

Rest calmly in this awareness and notice the vast spaciousness that opens up before you. Observe your mind, nature, your body, and even the sky floating by. Clouds come and go, thoughts come and go, sensations come and go.

With practice, as you invest the Seer with attention and awareness, all of the busyness and worries of the mind dissolve and you witness every object, feeling, and thought with a smile on your face.

To succeed, you must practice this exercise daily, the first thing in the morning, for 15 minutes.

> *Still your mind*
> *And all clouds disappear.*
> *Contemplate a single truth*
> *And clear sky appears.*
>
> — PATANJALI[2]

RADICAL FORGIVENESS

Every religion teaches the importance of forgiveness, whether in the form of turning the other cheek in Christianity or the Buddhist practice of sending loving-kindness to all beings. Yet it is very difficult to simply decide to forgive someone who has wronged you, and make the emotions of anger or the feeling of betrayal simply go away. It is equally difficult to forgive yourself and make the sense of shame or disappointment dissolve and no longer afflict you.

Sometimes we hold on so firmly to our resentments that we carry them with us to our deathbed. When we forgive ourselves and others, we can reprogram the toxic neural networks of our limbic brain. In order to truly forgive ourselves and others, we must upgrade the programming that is the source of our limiting beliefs. But we discover that there's a neurological catch-22: it is very difficult to create new neural networks until we practice forgiveness.

The following exercise was especially helpful to shamans after the Spanish Conquest of the Americas in the 15th to 16th centuries. With it, they were able to forgive the Conquistadors who wreaked havoc on their traditions and enslaved their people. In some parts of the Andes, this practice is known as "Burying the Sword of the Conquest." It works by re-imprinting the image of a loved one over the image of someone who has wronged you. This can help you override the programming of your prehistoric brain. It is not an easy practice, because the mind will resist holding the image of a loved one together with that of an enemy.

Exercise: Radical Forgiveness

This practice works best when you are relaxed.

Sit down comfortably and take a few deep, relaxing breaths. Call to your mind the image of a loved one, and feel the feelings of caring and affection. Hold this image for a count of three breaths. Now call to your mind the image of someone you feel has wronged you—a former lover or business partner, or someone who abused you physically or emotionally. For one long breath, feel the anger or resentment you have toward this person swelling up inside you. Now, for five long breaths, superimpose the image of your loved one over this person, and imagine how they blend and merge until only the image of your loved one remains, and only the feelings of love and caring endure.

This exercise must be repeated frequently for it to clear the toxic emotions and erase the neural networks in the limbic brain. You will notice that the intensity of your feelings of anger or resentment will gradually diminish, until one day you discover that they are extinguished. Then you will be able to draw the lesson that you still have to learn from that relationship and not have to waste time and energy on toxic emotions. Once we learn the lessons that our enemies have to teach us, we don't need to continue learning that way any longer.

DRAWING LIFE FROM YOUR DREAMS

Shamans believe that an enlightened person is one who not only recognizes truth but is able to bring forth truth in every situation he encounters. The enlightened person not only speaks truth but recognizes and understands the true nature of reality both when awake and when asleep.

Shamans believe that our waking reality is very similar to the world we experience during our sleeping dreams. This does not mean that the world is not real, that those are not real birds singing outside your window or real children playing at your feet or real neighbors bickering next door. The world is real, but our perception of that world is flawed. Our mind only ruffles the surface of the reality it observes, and thus perceives only its own distorted reflection. It therefore obscures the truth of a greater Reality.

Amazon sages speak of learning to dream with open eyes. They feel it is unfortunate that people in the West have stuffed dreaming time into the domain of sleep, where clouded consciousness inhibits recollections and blurs the images and insights that dreams are meant to reveal. Even when we recall dreams, the waking mind cannot grasp the few images that linger after many long hours of adventuring while asleep. The sages point out that the enlightened person is fully awake even while asleep, while the unenlightened human is fully asleep even while awake.

These sages believe that if we become lucid in our dreams, we can begin to change their tone and direction. Once we learn to change our sleeping dreams, we can begin to change our waking dreams. Then we begin to dream—awake and asleep—of our world with greater originality and lucidity. We guide our dreams to extraordinary domains where we learn from great teachers, visit distant lands, communicate (without electronic devices) with friends across the world, and meet with deceased ancestors.

Dreams are a part of our life, coming to us nightly, whether we are aware of them or not. They also come to us in the form of daydreams, a pastime for which many of us have been criticized for squandering time. But shamans respect their dreams—both of the nighttime and the daytime—because they contain messages from the spirit and the biosphere.

To draw life from your dreams, we recommend two exercises: Dream Yoga and Lucid Dreaming.

Through this Dream Yoga exercise, you will be able to better recall your dreams and will prepare yourself for the next exercise, Lucid Dreaming.

Exercise: Dream Yoga

Set your clock to awaken you five or ten minutes earlier than usual, ideally with gentle music rather than a radio talk show host or an alarming buzzer.

If you do not recall your dreams easily, try the following technique. Drink one half a glass of water before you go to bed and tell yourself, "When I wake up, I will drink the other half glass and remember my dreams."

Keep a notebook by the side of your bed, and when you wake up in the morning take a few moments to jot down keywords that will remind you of your dreams.

When you awaken, come out of your sleep slowly and luxuriously, basking in the afterglow of your dreams, relishing the flavors, scents, and images that linger in the early morning from your dreamtime adventures.

With your eyes closed, recall your dreams, and notice the urgency with which the waking mind wants to get on with the day's work, whether checking your e-mail, listening to the morning news, or getting ready for work. When you do open your eyes, do so gently.

Write what you recall in your dream journal, always using the present tense, as if you were still dreaming as you write, even if your dreams seem fuzzy or blurry at first. As you do this exercise, you might be amazed at how much more you recall as you write.

As soon as you wake up in the morning, drink the rest of the water and lie in bed with your eyes closed, allowing your dream images to flow back into awareness.

If you are likely to get up during the night to go to the bathroom, keep a recorder next to your bed and dictate the essentials of any interrupted dream.

■ ■ ■

Lucid dreaming is important because it helps us bring consciousness and awareness into our dreams. Once we learn lucid dreaming, dreams no longer just "happen" to us. As we realize we are dreaming, we are able to guide and direct our dreams.

Lucid dreaming is the first of three steps in the shaman's dream practices. The second is to bring awareness into your dreamless sleep, when you have no dream images in your awareness. The third is to bring your dreaming practice (not your dreams but the skill of dreaming) into your waking state, to understand that you are dreaming the world into being at all times.

Through lucid dreaming, shamans can agree to convene on a certain night at a place of power in nature. They may use a crystal or some other beautiful stone to facilitate their dream meeting. When they compare notes in the following days or weeks, they recognize that they had indeed shared the same *psychic space* and were able to recall what the others had said or done.

Exercise: Lucid Dreaming

Select a stone—perhaps a beautiful crystal—with no sharp edges and that fits nicely in the palm of your hands so that you can rub your hands together while holding it.

When you go to bed, set your intention to dream lucidly. For example, you might decide to dream about being in a mountain in the Himalayas, or perhaps a home you lived in during your childhood, or about visiting with relatives who are no longer living. You can also determine to visit a "university" where you will go to receive teaching and training.

As you concentrate, blow into your stone with a soft breath and ask your subconscious mind to bring the image of the stone into your dreams.

Hold the stone in your hand while you go to sleep.

During the night, the stone will fall out of your hand and end up somewhere in the bed. If you turn over and lie on it, you will likely surface from your deep sleep momentarily. Take the stone into your hands. Imagine that you are bringing it with you into your dreams, and reassert your intention to dream lucidly.

After a few tries, you will find that the stone will begin to appear in your dreams. You will realize that you are dreaming while you are in the dream. And, with time, you will become able to steer your dreams in your intended direction.

To succeed, you must practice this exercise daily.

WE ARE OUR STORIES

Shamans come from cultures where the written word has not yet replaced the storytelling tradition and where "facts" have not yet overthrown the myths and legends that express the soul of a people.

As nations and as individuals, we are the product of the stories we tell ourselves about our origins, our childhood, our life, and our close brushes with death. For example, for a long time, Christians believed that the story of Creation as told in the Bible was the only available explanation of how humans came to appear on the Earth. Then scientists discovered that there was another perspective, another story, and Darwinian evolution began to influence our culture's worldview. When we do not generate original stories of our own, we can easily adopt iterations of the generally accepted version of reality or the pop psychology themes of the time.

In our personal stories, we might feel hurt by rejection, for example when our first love was not reciprocated, or when we were told by our elementary school teacher that our drawing was "not worth saving" as she crumpled it up. Then, we have all experienced the loss of a loved one and feelings of being left alone to fend for ourselves in the world. When we see ourselves as victims in those tragic tales, we might turn that hurt or that loss into an apology for not being creative, or into an excuse for not "showing up" in our marriages and families. But when we are able to survive loss, defeat, abandonment, rejection, and failure and, instead, draw important lessons from those intense encounters with fate, then our stories become epics of great heroism in which we are the protagonist.

Everyone likes to think their tale is unlike anyone else's. We tend to invest hugely in the drama of our story, absolutely convinced not only that it is true but also that we ourselves are the product of our circumstances, but this is not the case.

■ ■ ■

Alberto:
I Am

My patients' stories are true. I know this because they have told me. They have invested their tale with sound and fury in an attempt to better understand their past. And each time, they recast the events of their past in a more convenient light, imposing 20/20 hindsight. The long-held story of being abused as a child, for example, explained timid and withdrawn adult behavior. The replayed story of a struggle with addiction explained not living up to full potential. These stories often served as an apology to life for what a person had become.

And I learned this lesson again as an anthropologist working with Amazon sages. The shamans believed that everything a person recalls about their past is a projection of an internal map held in their psyche.

"Amanda" was convinced she had been abandoned emotionally by her mother and father when she was very young. After many years in therapy, struggling with her abandonment issues, she went to a hypnotherapist who performed a hypnotic regression during which she saw vividly how her parents had abandoned her when she was 18 months old. After her session, Amanda confronted her mother—her father had already passed away by then. The mother explained that Amanda had been very colicky as a baby and, at that early age, both parents had gone on a weeklong holiday, leaving Amanda with her grandmother, who held her and cuddled her. The brain of the child, of course, did not recognize the parents' need for a little sleep but only realized that Mommy and Daddy had gone, perhaps never to come back.

Amanda taught me what the Amazon sages knew: namely, that trauma is not what actually happens but the way it is remembered—how it continues to live as a personal myth in the psyche. "A tale told by an idiot, full of sound and fury, signifying nothing," as Shakespeare said.

Only later would I understand the lesson of the shamans—and one of the primary lessons of this book: When you change the story, the world changes.

But, as you have heard—and it is well worth repeating—your story cannot be changed superficially by merely changing your mind or mentally altering the events of your childhood. For example, even after European maritime explorers sailed off the supposed "edge of the world" and came back to tell about it, proving that the world is round, many people continued to believe that that could not possibly be true, and they went on living as if the world were flat. The same skepticism occurred, even among the brightest minds of the time, after the discovery that the Earth orbits the sun.

You might wonder, then, what happened to Amanda upon hearing her mother's side of the story. Did that truth change the false belief that Amanda had created and fostered for so many years?

The shamans help clients change their stories at very deep layers of the psyche. There, it is possible to access and reprogram neural networks, but only after a close brush with illness or death or after a period of fasting, prayer, and preparation. Then, their clients can create a better tale, one in which they are cast as hero and not as victim.

Ideally, clients also discover they are the storytellers and not their stories, that they are the mythmakers and not the myths. This realization involves the prefrontal cortex, the only part of the brain that is able to attain this level of enlightened understanding and wield the brush to paint an entirely new landscape of our lives. And, yes, this is what Amanda did. But it took great effort on her part, as she went from being angry at her mother for abandoning her, to being angry at her mother for not abandoning her, to being angry at herself, to forgiving herself and embracing the great lessons she had received about being able to rely on herself always.

And now I want to tell you how I changed my story.

One time, I was in Canyon de Chelly in the American Southwest where I befriended an elderly medicine woman of the Navajo Nation. In the course of our conversation, this woman, "Charlotte," asked me who I was and about my family. I responded that I was born in Cuba; that, during my childhood, there was a terrible revolution where I saw much suffering; that, for political reasons, my father often had to leave us when I was a young boy; and that I had been raised without a positive role model for being a man.

The old woman smiled at me, and I felt it was my turn to ask her who she was and what she did. Her response took me back. She said, "The red-rock canyon walls am I, the desert wind am I, that child who did not eat today at the reservation am I."

And I thought to myself, what an interesting story, so much more interesting than mine, which I later understood had been shaped as much by my experience as by the pop psychology of the time. That very day I determined to change my story. I would no longer be the child who did not belong anywhere, wounded by a revolution that I was too young to fight in or flee from, and who required an older role model in order to become a man. But I discovered that I could not change my life story only by changing my mind about it, only by rationally determining to become someone different. No, I would need to transition from old-brain thinking to the wisdom of the prefrontal cortex, which means I would need to lay aside—even slay—my old mythologies and create new maps for the remainder of my journey.

Likewise, you can exchange your stories of scarcity, bereavement, loss, and suffering for a grander, more noble epic. You can be like Siddhartha, the young prince who left an easy but unfulfilling life in the palace to discover enlightenment and become the Buddha.

But, to change your story and rewire your brain, you have to quiet your HPA axis so that you can get out of fight-or-flight paralysis, stop responding to people and situations with anger and violence, and cease running away or hiding.

The sages of old knew that for a person to heal from trauma, that person had to discover a new personal mythology in which he or she ceased being the victim of a terrible childhood, a failed marriage, an illness, or of history itself. The shamans knew that person would need to paint a grand canvas and depict him- or herself as a heroic traveler and explorer.

When we understand that the stories of our lives both shape our neurology and are the product of neural networks, we can choose to change our stories in order to change our brains. Once we change our brains, we can start to have new and original experiences and craft more original stories from these. In this manner, like one hand washing the other, our experiences shape and mold our brain, and our brain shapes and informs our stories. We have two principal stories in our life: One is written in our genetic code, which many believe is fixed and immutable. The other is the psychological story (or stories) we consciously tell—and retell and retell and retell—ourselves. These stories are linked because often the chapters and verses of the latter are poorly edited versions of our parents' life and struggles.

The earlier exercise Reselecting Your Genetic Destiny will help you to rewrite your genetic tale. The following exercise will show you how to edit the story that defines your life journey.

■ ■ ■

Exercise: We Are Our Stories

Take a pen and paper and write a one-page fairy tale that starts with "Once upon a time . . . " Include a princess or prince, a warrior, and a dragon, but allow the story to unfold and gain in complexity as you weave in other characters and adventures. If you think this sounds childish, give yourself permission to be childlike for a few moments.

Now put this book down and try this exercise before you read further about the outcome of the practice.

Later today or tomorrow, select someone who will help you understand the significance of this fairy tale.

Read your story aloud to a friend or partner and look for themes. What genre is it: adventure, romance, a tale of despair, or a quest for love or fortune? Who is the main character: the princess, the dragon, the warrior, or another character?

Now change the tense from past to present and claim, for yourself, all actions of the primary character. For example, you might change "and then the king left the princess while her castle was being stormed" to "and then the king left me while my castle was being stormed."

Notice how the tone and significance of the story changes. This will reveal some of the beliefs inscribed in the primitive neural networks of your brain.

Now rewrite the story, casting your character as a hero or heroine who embarks upon a journey in search of meaning. For example, you change from "a princess who is abandoned by her family when her castle is under siege" to "a courageous maiden who follows her heart's calling to explore the world and discover her purpose in life, her reason for being, despite all the adversity she had to face."

As you rewrite your personal story, you may discover, for example, that your parents' divorce is not your story of abandonment but your opportunity to learn resilience and bravery early in life; that being unmarried is not your failure at love but an opportunity to develop your care and generosity toward others; that being humbled by life's circumstances is a chance to set aside pride and practice humility.

Then read your rewritten story as the parable it is. Identify with the lessons and gifts you experience in your life stories—and in your life.

And as you read, remember that your prefrontal cortex is laying pathways for your new neural networks of joy, inner peace, and enlightenment.

THE SHAMAN'S BATH

This is a very cleansing and healing bath formula. Repeat this bath as often as you like, especially on your day of fasting. Sage is used by shamans throughout the Americas to "smudge," or cleanse, the energy of a person or a place.

Recipe: The Shaman's Bath

½ cup baking soda
½ cup sea salt
10 drops of sage oil (essential oil)

Pour ingredients into a tub as you are filling it with warm water and soak your body for 20 minutes.
Rinse off.
Go straight to bed.

CHAPTER 14

THE POWER UP YOUR BRAIN PROGRAM

What you've read in *Power Up Your Brain* so far is the marriage of science and spirituality, of fact and tradition, of history and prehistory.

In the following pages, you will receive instructions regarding diet, fasting, dietary supplements, exercise, shamanic exercises, meditation, and imaging practices. The program entails five weeks of intensive practice, followed by a more moderate regular practice for maintenance.

You are about to embark on a journey toward enlightenment.

You will experience the benefits described throughout the earlier chapters in this book, specifically the creation of new neural pathways that will help you to heal from trauma and experience inner peace and enlightenment.

If possible, begin the Power Up Your Brain Program on the day of the full moon.

Important reminder: This Program involves fasting. Consult with your physician before engaging in this or any fasting program, especially if you are diabetic, have low blood sugar, take pharmaceutical medications, or are experiencing any physical condition that you believe you should discuss with your doctor or a professional health practitioner.

Week 1

During this week, you will begin a journey that will lead to significant changes in your body and profound experiences for your being. Depending on your lifestyle, you may not be aware of those changes, and you may even experience a certain amount of discomfort as your body begins to eliminate toxins.

Diet

Organics: Choose as many organic foods as are available. If finances are an issue, make sure to choose organic varieties of the following foods because they're most likely to be contaminated: apples, peaches, nectarines, pears, strawberries, cherries, imported grapes, celery, sweet bell peppers, spinach, lettuce, and potatoes.

Allergens: During this first week, modify your diet to reduce your consumption of foods that may contain allergens. The most common of these are foods that contain gluten—wheat, barley, and rye—as well as dairy products.

Totally eliminating gluten from your diet may be challenging, so you may wish to ask your doctor to perform a simple blood test to determine in advance if you are gluten sensitive. If the test is negative, meaning that you are not gluten sensitive, then there's no need to avoid gluten-containing foods.[1] An even better idea, which will serve you long after the Power Up Your Brain Program is completed, is to consider having a comprehensive blood evaluation for food allergies such as the Comprehensive Food Allergy Profile offered by Genova Diagnostics Laboratory. This simple blood evaluation will determine your unique level of sensitivity to 88 common foods.[2] The test provides a ranking of foods in terms of your sensitivity. We generally recommend that patients permanently remove all foods ranked at 2+ or 3+ from their diets and certainly throughout the rest of the Power Up Your Brain Program.

As much as possible, eliminate sugars and other simple carbohydrates such as highly refined flour. This means no pasta and breads made from processed flour. Instead choose products made from whole-grain flour, which you can purchase from health-food stores.

Fats: This is also the time to start focusing on the fats in your diet. While it may sound counterintuitive, dietary fats are *good* for the brain. This makes sense when you remember that some 70 percent of the brain is made of fat and that the source of this fat is your diet. So it's not so much the *amount* of fat that's in your diet, but the *type* of fat you consume that makes all the difference. Consuming foods made with hydrogenated, saturated fats not only builds a less functional brain that's at increased risk for diseases like Alzheimer's and Parkinson's, but will also compromise function day by day while increasing your risk for so many systemic diseases that are now epidemic in our society, like diabetes, depression, high blood pressure, and coronary artery disease. Now is the time to infuse your diet with sources of DHA and good fats like virgin organic olive oil, which may help protect the brain from Alzheimer's disease. New research now finds that oleocanthal, a compound found in virgin olive oil, modifies specific proteins called ADDLs that interfere with normal nerve function and may trigger memory loss. These modifications render the ADDLs less damaging to the brain.

Alcohol: While consuming one alcoholic drink per day for women and one to two drinks daily for men has been shown to reduce the risk for cognitive decline and even Alzheimer's disease, we recommend abstaining from alcohol during the first four weeks of the Power Up Your Brain Program.[3]

Caffeine: Discontinue caffeine. You will be able to reintroduce it later on.

Withdrawal Symptoms: If you have been aggressively consuming sugar, caffeine, or alcohol, you may experience significant withdrawal symptoms. The range of withdrawal symptoms is quite wide and can include everything from headaches, depression, fatigue, and mood swings to nausea, vomiting, insomnia, and fever depending on which substance you've given up.

To manage these symptoms, drink an additional eight-ounce glass of water two or three times daily, preferably spring water or reverse osmosis purified water, and meditate as described below. Accept that you may have to feel a little bit worse before you start feeling better.

Fasting

Do not fast during Week 1.

Dietary Supplements

Add the following natural supplements to your diet.

- **Vegetarian DHA:** 1,000 mg (milligrams) daily. Vegetarian DHA typically comes in the form of a 200 mg capsule, so take five capsules daily, all at once or split the dose throughout the day, with or without food. Keep refrigerated.

- **Olive oil, virgin, organic:** 1 tablespoon daily. This may be added to salad dressing, drizzled over steamed vegetables, combined with freshly juiced organic vegetables, or consumed with whole-grain bread. The oil must be consumed uncooked, so olive oil used in cooking does not count toward this requirement.

- **Alpha-lipoic acid, controlled release:** 600 mg daily, 30 minutes before meals or on empty stomach. Available under the brand name ALAmax CR from www.Xymogen.com (tel. 800-647-6100).

- **Coconut oil, virgin, organic:** 1 tablespoon each morning. Feel free to add this to a smoothie or use it as a spread on whole-grain bread. Alternatively, capsules of coconut oil are now available.

- **Pterostilbene** (pronounced *tero-STILL-bean*): 50 mg each morning and evening, with or without food.*

- **Sulforaphane:** 30 mg each morning and evening, with or without food.*

- **Curcumin from turmeric extract:** 200 mg each morning and evening, with or without food.*

- **Green tea extract:** 200 mg each morning and evening, with or without food.*

*These supplements are contained in 1 capsule of Nrf2 Activator, available from Xymogen: 800-647-6100 or www.Xymogen.com. Nrf2 Activator also contains BioPerine, a pepper extract that significantly enhances the absorption of the active components of this unique supplement.

Physical Exercise

Ask your physician to help you determine your exercise tolerance.

Aerobics: Exercise (walk, bike, or jog) at a sustained aerobic pace for 20 minutes every day—or more if you're in good physical condition. Set your target pulse rate at a number equal to 180 minus your age, unless your doctor advises otherwise. Don't include warm-up or cool-down times in this 20-minute total.

If you are inclined, purchase a wristwatch-type monitoring device such as the Polar Heart Rate Monitor, which will give you an instantaneous readout of your pulse. These devices are available at most sporting goods stores and online.

Yoga/Stretching: Practice yoga or a similar stretching/flexibility program at least twice a week for at least 30 minutes per session.

Shamanic Exercises

The Shaman's Bath: Enjoy this once a week, on the day of your choice, in the evening before going to bed.

Quieting Your HPA Axis: Perform this exercise twice each week in the evening before going to bed.

Meditation

Participate in the Power Up Your Brain Program's daily Planetary Meditation. Download this peace meditation—along with an image that can be used as your desktop screen saver—from www.PowerUpYourBrain.com. As you do the meditation, try to tune in with others around the planet who are meditating at the same time.

Relationships

Reflect on your relationships with yourself and others, especially people who are important to you. Think about who these people are and how you reaching out to them today. How are you celebrating the ones you love? How are you honoring yourself?

Contemplate your interconnectedness with all human beings and with all creatures of the Earth. As you prepare to eat a meal, say a short prayer of blessing and imagine all the different plants, animals, and people who have contributed to your nourishment. Include not only the farmers, growers, and livestock raisers but also the handlers, truckers, and grocers.

Week 2 Through Week 4

As you move forward from Week 2 through Week 4, you may experience a heightened awareness of your being, a greater appreciation for yourself, and a diminishing amount of anxiety and anger in your life. As you smile at the person who just cut in front of you in the grocery checkout line, you are a step closer toward an enlightened life.

Diet

Continue to choose as many organic foods as are available.

Continue to avoid allergens, hydrogenated and saturated fats, alcohol, and caffeine.

Fruits & Vegetables: Eat at least five to six servings of fresh fruits and vegetables daily. When fresh produce isn't available, choose frozen preparations over canned.

Carbohydrates: Reduce your intake of carbohydrates to one serving per day—two slices of whole-grain bread or one serving of whole-grain pasta, or cereal (unless you exercise strenuously, in which case your body will need increased amounts of complex carbohydrates, like whole-grain cereals, pastas, or breads).

Fasting

You will fast twice in this part of the Power Up Your Brain Program: once during Week 2 and once during Week 3.

Choose a day to fast.

If you began the program on the day of the full moon, then the fourth day of this second week will be the 11th day after the full moon and will correspond to the ideal fasting and meditation day, as described in the Ayurvedic texts (as mentioned in Chapter 12); this will synchronize your fasting and deepen your meditative experience as you energetically connect with others who also adopt this program.

If you are not able to fast on the fourth day of the second week, then choose a day when you have no demanding business or personal obligations.

Fast again during Week 3, ideally one week after your first fast.

Do not fast during Week 4.

On the days you fast, drink ample amounts of water.

If you find fasting to be an overwhelming challenge, eat fresh fruit, such as sliced oranges, on the day you fast. Again, it's important to check with your physician before engaging in a fasting program, especially if you are diabetic, have low blood sugar, take pharmaceutical medications, or are experiencing any other physical concerns.

Dietary Supplements

Follow the same recommendations as in Week 1.

On the fasting day, continue to take all of your nutritional supplements, but add a second tablespoon of coconut oil and a second tablespoon of olive oil in the afternoon. Take a double dosage of pterostilbene, sulforaphane, curcumin (from turmeric extract), and green tea extract twice on this day only; or simply take two capsules of Nrf2 Activator morning and evening.

Physical Exercise

Practice yoga or a similar stretching/flexibility program at least twice a week for at least 30 minutes per session.

Increase your daily aerobic workout to 30 minutes, if possible.

Refrain from aerobic exercise on the day you fast.

Shamanic Exercises

Open and close your shamanic exercises with the Creating Sacred Space prayer, or a similar prayer of your own creation or choosing.

Sky Gazing: Perform this exercise each morning at sunrise.

Dream Yoga and Lucid Dreaming: Perform these exercises each evening.

Quieting Your HPA Axis: Perform this exercise two times a week, in the evening before going to bed.

Reselecting Your Genetic Destiny: Perform this meditation once each week.

We Are Our Stories: Perform once during the week and develop your new life story, your personal mythology in which you are the hero.

Shaman's Bath: Enjoy this once each week in the evening before going to bed.

Meditation

Participate in the Power Up Your Brain Program's daily Planetary Meditation. Download this peace meditation—along with an image that can be used as your desktop screen saver—from www.PowerUpYourBrain.com. As you do the meditation, try to tune in with others around the planet who are meditating at the same time.

Often during each day, take time to be consciously aware of your breath in order to cultivate stillness. Take long, deep breaths and feel the air move in and out of your body. Notice the sensations in your body as you breathe. And as your breathing becomes more rhythmic, you will find your sense of inner peace growing.

Relationships

Eliminate toxic relationships. Make a list of the people you need to forgive, and employ the Radical Forgiveness practice in Chapter 13.

Week 5

In Week 5, you will continue your hero's journey with greater awareness of and appreciation for yourself and your being. You are on your way to enlightenment.

As you eliminate toxins in your body and your brain, you will notice that your senses become more refined: colors become sharper, feelings become deeper and clearer, and your other senses, including touch, hearing, and smell, may become heightened. You will find that situations that once caused you stress or duress can now be dealt with much more elegantly and gracefully. As your brain becomes clearer, your meditation becomes easier. The noise level in your head is reduced greatly.

Diet

Continue to choose as many organic foods as are available.

Continue to avoid allergens, hydrogenated and saturated fats, and caffeine.

Continue to eat an elevated number of whole fruits and vegetables—at least five to six servings.

Continue consuming only one serving of carbohydrates per day.

Alcohol: You may consume alcohol if you wish, preferably organic red wine. Drink, at most, one glass with your evening meal, at most three times during this week. Do not consume alcohol on the fasting day.

Calorie Consumption: Implement calorie reductions or, if you are already consuming calories at the recommended level, make no changes—do not restrict your calorie consumption any further.

Women: reduce daily calorie consumption to 2,000 calories, or as advised by your physician.

Men: reduce daily calorie consumption to 2,550 calories, or as advised by your physician.

Remember that these are only general recommendations. Consult your physician or dietician for specific recommendations based upon your height, level of activity, muscularity, metabolism, underlying medical conditions, medications, and other factors.

Fasting

You will fast for one day during this week.

If possible, choose the 11th day after the full moon, which is the ideal fasting and meditation day, and it will synchronize your fasting and deepen your meditation experience as you energetically connect with others who also adopt this program.

Dietary Supplements

Follow the same recommendations as in Week 1.

On the fasting day, continue to take all of your nutritional supplements, but add a second tablespoon of coconut oil and a second tablespoon of olive oil in the afternoon. Take a double dosage of pterostilbene, sulforaphane, curcumin (from turmeric extract), and green tea extract twice on this day only; or simply take two capsules of Nrf2 Activator morning and evening.

Physical Exercise

Practice yoga or a similar stretching/flexibility program at least twice a week for at least 30 minutes per session.

Reduce your exercise from daily workouts to five days a week, but increase each workout to 40 to 45 minutes, if possible.

Coincide your exercise-free day with your fasting day.

Shamanic Exercises

Open and close your shamanic exercises with the Creating Sacred Space prayer, or a similar prayer of your own creation or choosing.

Perform the Sky Gazing exercise each morning at sunrise.

Perform the Dream Yoga and Lucid Dreaming exercises each evening.

Perform the Quieting Your HPA Axis exercise twice during this week in the evening before going to bed.

Enjoy a Shaman's Bath once each week in the evening before going to bed.

Meditation

Participate in the Power Up Your Brain Program's daily Planetary Meditation. Download the daily image as your desktop screen saver, and tune in to the Human Global Matrix of others around the planet who are meditating at the same time.

Often during each day, be aware of your breath and cultivate stillness.

Relationships

Ask for forgiveness of anyone you may have wronged. Drop them a handwritten note in the mail, or get on the telephone with them and say you are sorry directly. "I'm sorry" is one of the most powerful sentences that our higher brain knows. Then continue to work on forgiving anyone who you believe has wronged you, using the Radical Forgiveness exercise in Chapter 13.

Thereafter

Now, after five weeks in the Power Up Your Brain Program, you are well on your journey toward a healed brain, one that is increasingly free of the damaging effects of stress and trauma, and that is primed for enlightenment.

Diet

Continue to choose as many organic foods as are available.

Continue to avoid allergens and hydrogenated and saturated fats.

Continue to eat an elevated number of whole fruits and vegetables, at least five to six servings.

Continue consuming only one serving of carbohydrates each day and up to one glass of wine daily (if desired), but not on your fasting day.

Continue on your restricted calorie eating plan. Women can have up to 2,000 calories per day, and men can have up to 2,550 calories. Remember that these are only general recommendations. Consult your physician or dietician for specific recommendations.

Caffeine: Reintroduce caffeine in the form of coffee or tea, if you wish. Consume no more than 60 mg of caffeine each day, preferably in the morning.

Read labels. A typical 8-ounce cup of brewed coffee will contain from 60 to 120 mg of caffeine, depending on the type and how finely it is ground. Green tea contains a predictable 20 mg of caffeine in an 8-ounce cup. Black tea contains 45 mg in an 8-ounce cup.

Monitor your response to caffeine carefully. Reduce the amount if symptoms of overstimulation, such as insomnia, follow caffeine use.

Fasting

Continue to fast one day a month, preferably on the 11th day after the full moon.

Dietary Supplements

Continue to take your nutritional supplements.

On the days you fast, increase your daily supplements, as described on page 181.

Physical Exercise

Practice yoga or a similar stretching/flexibility program at least twice a week for at least 30 minutes per session.

Continue to do aerobic exercise for 40 to 45 minutes, 5 days a week. Refrain from aerobic exercise on the day of your fast.

Shamanic Exercises

Continue with the shamanic exercises: Creating Sacred Space, Sky Gazing, Dream Yoga, Lucid Dreaming, Quieting Your HPA Axis, and the Shaman's Bath.

Meditation

Participate in the Power Up Your Brain Program's daily Planetary Meditation. Download this peace meditation—along with an image that can be used as your desktop screen saver—from www.PowerUpYourBrain.com. As you do the meditation, try to tune in with others around the planet who are meditating at the same time.

Often during each day, take time to be consciously aware of your breath in order to cultivate stillness. Take long, deep breaths and feel the air move in and out of your body. Notice the sensations in your body as you breathe. And as your breathing becomes more rhythmic, you will find your sense of inner peace growing.

Relationships

Cultivate relationships with people that uplift and inspire you. Choose your friends carefully, and care for them like a gardener tends to his flowers. Invest prime time and energy into the friendships that you want to take with you for the rest of your life.

Week 1

Diet

- *Organics:* Choose
- *Allergens:* Reduce
- *Fats:* Avoid hydrogenated, saturated
- *Alcohol:* Avoid
- *Caffeine:* Avoid
- *Fruits & vegetables:* No change from normal
- *Carbohydrates:* No change from normal
- *Calorie consumption:* No change from normal
- *Fasting:* No fasting this week

Dietary Supplements

- *Vegetarian DHA:* 1,000 mg daily
- *Olive oil:* 1 tbsp daily
- *Alpha-lipoic acid:* 600 mg daily, 30 minutes before meals
- *Coconut oil:* Virgin, organic; 1 tbsp in morning
- *Pterostilbene*:* 50 mg morning & evening
- *Sulforaphane*:* 30 mg morning & evening
- *Curcumin*:* 200 mg morning & evening
- *Green tea extract*:* 200 mg morning & evening

*Note: These are all contained in 1 capsule of Nrf2 Activator, available from Xymogen.

Physical Exercise

- *Aerobic:* 20 minutes daily
- *Yoga/Stretch:* At least twice a week

Shamanic Exercises

- *Quieting Your HPA Axis:* Twice during the week before bed
- *Shaman's Bath:* Once during the week at the end of the day

Meditation

- *Planetary Meditation:* Daily

Relationships

- Celebrate those close to you, and yourself
- Imagine the interconnectedness of all beings on Earth

Weeks 2–4	
Diet	
• *Organics:* Choose • *Allergens:* Avoid • *Fats:* Avoid hydrogenated, saturated • *Alcohol:* Avoid • *Caffeine:* Avoid	• *Fruits & vegetables:* Increase • *Carbohydrates:* Reduce to 1 serving per day • *Calorie consumption:* No change from normal • *Fasting:* Once during the week in Weeks 2 and 3; no fasting in Week 4
Dietary Supplements	
• *Vegetarian DHA:* 1,000 mg daily • *Olive oil:* 1 tbsp daily, plus 1 additional tbsp on fasting day • *Alpha-lipoic acid:* 600 mg daily, 30 minutes before meals • *Coconut oil:* Virgin, organic; 1 tbsp in morning, plus 1 additional tbsp on fasting day	• *Pterostilbene*:* 50 mg morning & evening; double this on fasting day • *Sulforaphane*:* 30 mg morning & evening; double this on fasting day • *Curcumin*:* 200 mg morning & evening; double this on fasting day • *Green tea extract*:* 200 mg morning & evening; double this on fasting day
*Note: These are all contained in 1 capsule of Nrf2 Activator, available from Xymogen.	
Physical Exercise	
• *Aerobic:* 30 minutes daily; do not exercise on fasting day	• *Yoga/Stretch:* At least twice a week; not on fasting day

Shamanic Exercises	
• *Creating Sacred Space:* Daily before other shamanic exercises • *Quieting Your HPA Axis:* Twice during the week in the evening • *Reselecting Your Genetic Destiny:* Once during the week	• *Shaman's Bath:* Once during the week at the end of the day • *Sky Gazing:* Daily at sunrise • *Dream Yoga:* Daily • *Lucid Dreaming:* Daily • *We Are Our Stories:* Once during the week
Meditation	
• *Planetary Meditation:* Daily	• *Breath Awareness:* Often
Relationships	
• Eliminate toxic relationships	• Practice Radical Forgiveness

Week 5

Diet

• *Organics:* Choose • *Allergens:* Avoid • *Fats:* Favor low carbohydrate, low saturated fat • *Alcohol:* Red wine, 1 glass 3 times per week, if desired (not on fasting day)	• *Caffeine:* Avoid • *Fruits & vegetables:* Increase • *Carbohydrates:* 1 serving per day • *Calorie consumption:* Women reduce to 2,000 daily; Men reduce to 2,550 daily • *Fasting:* Once during the week

Dietary Supplements

• *Vegetarian DHA:* 1,000 mg daily • *Olive oil:* 1 tbsp daily, plus 1 additional tbsp on fasting day • *Alpha-lipoic acid:* 600 mg daily, 30 minutes before meals • *Coconut oil:* Virgin, organic; 1 tbsp in morning, plus 1 additional tbsp on fasting day	• *Pterostilbene*:* 50 mg morning & evening; double this on fasting day • *Sulforaphane*:* 30 mg morning & evening; double this on fasting day • *Curcumin*:* 200 mg morning & evening; double this on fasting day • *Green tea extract*:* 200 mg morning & evening; double this on fasting day

*Note: These are all contained in 1 capsule of Nrf2 Activator, available from Xymogen.

Physical Exercise

• *Aerobic:* 40–45 minutes, 5 days; not on fasting day	• *Yoga/Stretch:* At least twice a week; not on fasting day

Shamanic Exercises	
• *Creating Sacred Space:* Prior to other shamanic exercises • *Quieting Your HPA Axis:* Twice during the week in the evening	• *Shaman's Bath:* Once during the week at the end of the day • *Sky Gazing:* Daily at sunrise • *Dream Yoga:* Daily • *Lucid Dreaming:* Daily
Meditation	
• *Planetary Meditation:* Daily	• *Breath Awareness:* Often
Relationships	
• Ask for forgiveness	• Forgive using Radical Forgiveness

Thereafter	
Diet	
• *Organics:* Choose • *Allergens:* Avoid • *Fats:* Favor low carbohydrate, low saturated fat • *Alcohol:* Red wine, 1 glass 3 times per week, if desired (not on fasting day)	• *Caffeine:* Coffee or tea, max 60 mg daily, if desired • *Fruits & vegetables:* Increase • *Carbohydrates:* 1 serving per day • *Calorie consumption:* Women reduce to 2,000 daily; Men reduce to 2,550 daily • *Fasting:* Once during the week
Dietary Supplements	
• *Vegetarian DHA:* 1,000 mg daily • *Olive oil:* 1 tbsp daily, plus 1 additional tbsp on fasting day • *Alpha-lipoic acid:* 600 mg daily, 30 minutes before meals • *Coconut oil:* Virgin, organic; 1 tbsp in morning, plus 1 additional tbsp on fasting day	• *Pterostilbene*:* 50 mg morning & evening; double this on fasting day • *Sulforaphane*:* 30 mg morning & evening; double this on fasting day • *Curcumin*:* 200 mg morning & evening; double this on fasting day • *Green tea extract*:* 200 mg morning & evening; double this on fasting day
*Note: These are all contained in 1 capsule of Nrf2 Activator, available from Xymogen.	

Physical Exercise	
• *Aerobic:* 40–45 minutes, 5 days; not on fasting day	• *Yoga/Stretch:* At least twice a week; not on fasting day

Shamanic Exercises	
• *Creating Sacred Space:* Prior to other shamanic exercises • *Quieting Your HPA Axis:* As necessary • *Shaman's Bath:* Once during the week at the end of the day	• *Sky Gazing:* Daily at sunrise • *Dream Yoga:* Daily • *Lucid Dreaming:* Daily

Meditation	
• *Planetary Meditation:* Daily	• *Breath Awareness:* Often

Relationships
• Cultivate relationships with people who uplift and inspire you

CHAPTER 15

SEARCHING FOR
YOUR SOUL

The search for the soul has preoccupied humans for centuries. At first, our ancestors thought the soul had its seat in the heart; later, numerous other organs, including the liver and the spleen, became candidates for housing the soul. Eventually, when we could not find the soul in any of these locations, we decided that it must reside in the head, inside the brain. Yet the ancient Egyptians had little use for the brain: while they carefully mummified all of a deceased person's organs, they drained the brain by inserting straws through the nasal passage into the cranial cavity and tossed the whole bloody mess away.

Today, most scientists would argue that what we call consciousness is an epiphenomenon, or secondary by-product, of the brain—that is, that the neural circuitry in the brain creates consciousness. In fact, Francis Crick, one of the discoverers of DNA, states in his book *The Astonishing Hypothesis: The Scientific Search for the Soul* that everything to be learned about the soul can be found by studying the workings of the human brain. In contrast, shamans are more prone to believe the reverse, that the brain is an epiphenomenon of consciousness, and that consciousness itself utilizes complex evolutionary mechanisms to create the neural circuitry that allows us to become aware of ourselves and the universe.

Perhaps someday we will discover that *both* modern scientists and ancient shamans and mystics were right. Perhaps scientists will discover that, indeed, we are more than a sack of neurons, and perhaps mystics will discover that the brain and the body are both essential elements of consciousness. But what if we did not have to wait for leading scientists and spiritual leaders to pass a verdict on this matter? What if we were to conduct the experiment ourselves?

IN THE BEGINNING WAS THE WORD

Science provides answers to the great questions that once could only be answered by religion. When these scientific answers are first discovered, they seem like heresies to the established order. We once believed the world had been created 6,000 years ago, that the Earth was flat, and that our blue-green planet was the center of the universe. When Galileo tried to describe the science behind Copernicus's discovery that the Earth revolved around the sun, he was sentenced to house arrest for his heresy. Yet, today, everyone accepts that fact that the Earth is not the center of the universe.

Many religions teach that we have a soul that is eternal and undying, even though our physical bodies eventually return to dust. Materialistic scientists would argue that of course, energy and matter cannot be destroyed, and every particle in our bodies will be recycled into rivers, eagles, or cosmic dust.

But the shaman believes that it is possible for each one of us to have the experience of an eternal aspect of ourselves.

■ ■ ■

Alberto:
Think with Your Heart, Feel with Your Head

I remember the first time I held a human brain in my hands. My friend Brian, a student in medical school, had invited me to join him that evening while he removed the brain from a cadaver that he and his dissection partner had been working on. Brian had the brain to himself, as his partner had passed on the experience, saying that she was going into obstetrics and had little interest in that part of the human anatomy.

The double door at the University of California Anatomy Laboratory was a ponderous, institutional gray. The sound of its bar lock ricocheted off cold linoleum. The room was the size of a small warehouse and blue-gray bright with fluorescent light. There were four rows of Bakelite-topped tables upon which vague shapes were draped with black rubberized sheets. The stench of formalin wrinkled my nose. Brian set a stainless steel hacksaw beside a bucket of Kentucky Fried Chicken and an empty beer bottle, then slid off the tall stool at the head of his table.

Brian's cadaver was that of a young woman. The rubber sheet had been folded back to expose her upper chest, neck, and head. Her skin was like a calf's hide, her complexion gray and tinged with olive drab.

"This is Jennifer," Brian said. "We've been together all semester." *He lifted the surgical saw. "She's taught me more about the human body than I knew there was to learn. I'll never forget her."*

"Brian—"

"Tonight she is going to lose her head for me, and I wanted you to be here."

"Thanks."

His eyes held mine in a matter-of-fact stare.

"You don't get to see a decapitation these days without a hundred-grand student loan and a year's worth of medical school. I thought you'd be interested."

"Why?"

"Psychologist."

"Yeah," I said. "When people lose their heads, they come to me."

He stared at me for a second, trying to gauge my tone of voice.

"You don't have to do this if you don't want to," he said. "I just thought—I mean, if you're uncomfortable . . ."

"It's all right," I said.

"If you'd rather . . ."

I looked at the bucket of chicken. "I'm just trying to stay away from fried foods," I said. I wasn't prepared to admit that I was strangely revolted, yet irresistibly fascinated, by the body on the table. He handed me a beer.

"Eat afterward?" he said.

"If we can."

"Incredible, huh? Just down the hall, there's a lab where they conduct the foremost research in recombinant DNA. One floor down, neurologists are teaming up with biochemists and computer gurus to simulate the neural pathways of simple brain functions. But here we are cutting up dead people just like Leonardo da Vinci did five hundred years ago." He looked around the room at all the black-draped figures.

"We start on the back," he said, "because it takes a while to get used to what you're doing, and it's easier if you don't have to look at the face—as if they can really look back at you and make you feel guilty for violating them with a scalpel."

He reached down and cupped the cadaver's chin in the palm of his hand. Her head moved back slightly. Decisively, he placed the serrated blade of the saw on a wedge of cartilage between the exposed vertebrae of her neck. I couldn't take my eyes from it. When the head was free from the body, he held it in both hands. While we talked, he took what looked like a large dental drill from a drawer, plugged it into an electrical socket, and selected a bit, a round, disklike blade about two inches in diameter.

"They save the best for last," he said, and the handpiece whirred. "Hold her for me, will you?"

I took the head in my hands and positioned it for him, and he brought the spinning blade down on the forehead. When he was through, when he had rotated the head a full 360 degrees, he switched off the little saw. The whine of the blade still rang in my ears. There was a curious smell in the air, and a fine powder of bone dust lay on the face and clung to its eyelashes. He leaned over and gently blew it away.

"Imagine," he said. "No human being has ever seen Jennifer's brain. You and I are the first. Drum roll, maestro."

And he pulled the calavarium away from the skull. I had seen a human brain. I had seen many, floating in formalin-filled lab jars. But that moment will always live for me.

Aristotle thought that the brain cooled the blood, that thinking was a function of the heart. Rene Descartes described the brain as the pump of a nerve fountain. It has been compared to a clock, a telephone switchboard, a computer; yet the mechanics of the brain are far more intricate than any analog. Theorist Lyall Watson wrote that if the brain were so simple that we could understand it, we would be so simple that we couldn't. And the source of all this theory and speculation was the walnut-shaped, fleshy, gray mass of tissue before me.

Brian looked at me and nodded his head toward Jennifer's. Once again, I placed a hand on either side of her face, and Brian eased the brain from her head. He stood weighing it in his hands for a moment, then handed it to me. It was heavy.

Brian interrupted the silence. "I don't believe it either," he said.[1]

That evening, I took with me a tiny portion of Jennifer's brain that we had sliced and diced and placed on a glass slide, the kind you use in a microscope. I said to myself that I wanted to "look inside her head" more carefully at a later date. The slide contained a small piece of Jennifer's prefrontal cortex.

Weeks later, I was in Cuzco, the capital of the ancient Inca empire and the longest continually inhabited city in the Americas. The ancestors of the Inca had built the original mud-and-straw structures, and the Inca had built great stone palaces on top of them. I was visiting Don Antonio Morales, my translator and informant as I investigated the healers and sages of the Andes, and whom I would later discover was one of the great shamans in the area. That night, when I entered Don Antonio's simple cabin, the first thing he said to me was, "You've brought someone with you." I immediately replied that I had come alone, but he gazed beyond me to the back of the room, and he said that the guest that I had brought had come uninvited. And then he began to describe Jennifer to me, how she had lived, whom she had loved, and how she had died.

The hair on the back of my neck stood on end. I was not used to having uninvited guests accompany me, but I recalled that I had been sleeping restlessly since that experience with Brian in the anatomy laboratory. And now this old sage was telling me that Jennifer's soul had attached itself to me.

"It's because you are warm-hearted and compassionate," the old man said. "Although she had died, her soul was caught between the world of the living and the world of spirit. She was trapped in a nightmare that she could not wake up from. And perhaps she knew, somewhere deep inside, that you would bring her to me and that we would relieve her suffering."

The old man pointed out that Jennifer's soul had become attached to an object of hers that I had removed without permission. I immediately started digging through my backpack and pulled out the microscope slide.

"What is it?" Don Antonio asked.

"It's her brain, a piece of it," I said.

He looked at me and frowned. "You've done a very bad thing," he said. "But maybe it was for the best. Now we will heal her and help her go back home to the world of spirit."

Thus began my training with the shamans. Since then, I have had a direct and palpable experience of my own soul and the beauty of the souls of others around me. I have discovered the soul to be the finest aspect of human nature, that part of us that finds beauty everywhere regardless of how much ugliness there is around us. It is the part of us that no longer searches for the truth but, rather, brings truth to every encounter. It is the part of us that no longer seeks happiness but infuses every instant with joy. It is the part of us that practices kindness and lives in simplicity.

The shamans believe that the soul is all that is beautiful and noble about being human. The soul has the possibility of becoming eternal because beauty and nobility are eternal. But to experience this, we first have to heal the trauma and pain from our past and become enlightened.

The great experiment that each one of us can perform is to recover an essential aspect of ourselves that we have lost as a result of pain, trauma, and stress. In metaphorical terms, this is the part of ourselves that never left the Garden of Eden, that still walks with beauty in the world, connected to the rivers and the trees, and that speaks with God easily and readily. We believe that the key to this lies above our eyebrows, in our prefrontal cortex. Once this brain is awakened, we can experience brain synergy and understand who we are and what we want from life.

EPILOGUE

Alberto Villoldo:
The Seer's Reward

Third day of fasting. I am on the southern slope, below the ruins of Machu Picchu, in a temple cave that archeologists have not yet restored. Abandoned cultivation terraces that once fed an entire citadel now lie in ruins above and below where I am camped. The refined Inca stonework is evident in the back of the cave, and after cutting down the tall grass, I was able to arrange a comfortable spot for myself, protected from the sun and rain. This morning I found a snake, which had obviously been warming itself all night from my body heat, coiled by the foot of my sleeping bag. I am not sure which one of us was more startled, yet the snake was still lethargic, as it had been a chilly night, and I was able to coax it out of the cave with a stick. I am certain that this is its cave, that I was the intruder, but there was no arguing over this. For two more days, it would be my cave.

Yesterday was sheer torture. The groaning of my empty stomach was nowhere near as bad as the torment of my mind. I would try to meditate, but could not stop salivating every time my thoughts wandered to the chocolate bar I had stashed away at the bottom of my backpack, to the taste of the warm chocolate, and how every cell in my body longed for

the fortifying sugar and cacao. Finally, toward sunset, I tore through my
pack and found the object of my torture, opened the foil wrapper, and
tossed the bar to the Urubamba River below.

What a relief. Now I only had the rumbling in my belly to worry
about. . .

— Alberto's Journal[1]

Someone once explained to me that the difference between religion and science is that in science, you come up with a hypothesis and you test it out against the facts. If the facts don't support your theory, you toss it out and come up with a better one. If your assumption is that stones fall upward, and the facts prove you wrong, then you have to come up with a better premise. By contrast, in religion, if the facts don't support your hypothesis, you dismiss the evidence until better proof is offered, because religion is the realm of faith, not facts. Faith has rallied men and women to heroic acts and inspired them to great works of art. Facts have seldom moved the soul or the imagination.

With religion, the older the better. There are few new religions. With science, the newer the better. Both the physics and the medicine of 20 years ago are dated, yet the religions of hundreds of years ago remain vibrant and alive. For shamans, old and new, past and present, all collapse into the eternal moment. Neither science nor religion, shamanism is based neither on proof or belief. It is based on experience.

Shamans, yogis, and mystics around the planet devised a series of experiments in consciousness that anyone willing to put the effort and time into the research could replicate. The experiment was elegantly simple: *Quiet the mind and discover the Seer within.* Once you discover the Seer, when you are able to drop in between the moments, when the clock stops ticking and you have not died, then you can experience infinity and become a master of your own destiny.

And while the Seers were often the men and women who were able to interpret what the crack in the turtle's shell meant for the emperor's future or where the bison where going to be the following morning, this was considered an outer manifestation of a deeper gift. The reward that the Seer discovered when he turned his gaze within was the understanding of the workings of Creation and his role in the unfolding of a heavenly design.

The master shamans of the Andes, refer to this as the "wisdom that can be known but not told." I am not a good enough poet to express the freedom and joy one attains as a result of discovering the Seer. The experience is there for all who are willing to try it. And it is as old as humanity itself. But it requires taming the great beast of toxic emotions, a creature as fearsome as the chocolate bar that obsessed me in the Amazon, as terrifying as a many-headed serpent like the fabled Hydra that Hercules struggled against, for each time he cut off one of its heads, two more would grow back.

The shamanic exercises in *Power Up Your Brain* are among the most effective and powerful that I know. When combined with the recommended brain nutrients, dietary recommendations, fasting, calorie reduction, and physical exercise, they will help you heal from trauma and discover a newfound inner peace and creativity. They will allow you to take part in the most ancient experience in human consciousness.

We invite you to try the program and take your brain out for a spin to see what it can do. But first, you must get rid of the chocolate in your mind, throw the internal chatterbox of disturbing emotions into the river, push the lethargic snakes of interruption away from under your feet. Take up the Power Up Your Brain Program, and after you have tried it, let us know how well it is working!

■ ■ ■

David Perlmutter:
The Most Powerful Medicine of All

We stand at the threshold of the next quantum leap in human evolution. For the first time in the history of all living things on the planet, a species will now take an active and conscious role in directing its genetic destiny. Evolution, until now, has been stepwise and compliant with Darwinian doctrine. In a sense, even self-directed evolution, as we have described, is Darwinian, since choosing to pursue its constructs represents a "natural selection" process.

The ultimate goal of amplification of neurogenesis and enhancing neuroplasticity, utilizing the dietary and lifestyle modifications recommended in this text, is to create a fertile garden to enhance the effectiveness of the meditation programs described. And over the past two years, as this project unfolded, my task was pretty much focused on the former, while Alberto, with his rich experiences living and working with shamans in the Andes, was perfectly suited for the latter.

As we progressed on the project, however, Alberto and I noted how we gravitated to a more central common ground as I began incorporating meditative recommendations into the practice of neurology, and he began to embrace the technology and nutritional approaches that have become central to my medical practice.

With the thought of fully combining our two seemingly disparate approaches, we offered a weeklong intensive therapy program in Naples, Florida, whereby patients were trained in deep and focused shamanic practices while, at the same time, being treated with aggressive, high-tech approaches to enhance brain function and receptivity. The latter included both hyperbaric oxygen therapy and intravenous administration of glutathione.

What transpired was life-changing not only for the participants but for Alberto and me as well. Individuals who were struggling with lifelong issues were finally able to gain the necessary insight to understand and redirect many of their deep-seated and maladaptive responses.

Clearly, the whole of the program proved much greater than the simple sum of the parts. And these achievements have served to support the development of our programs at our respective facilities: the Center for Energy Medicine in Chile and the Perlmutter Health Center in Naples, Florida. Enhancing antioxidant protection, detoxification, growth of mitochondria, and reduction of inflammation by the implementation of the techniques described in the Power Up Your Brain Program provide health benefits far beyond enhancing brain function and enriching the meditative experience. Inflammation, excessive action of free radicals, and toxicity represent pathological biochemistry that underpins a vast array of health issues, including coronary artery disease, cancer, arthritis, diabetes, asthma, inflammatory bowel disease, and autism. And beyond maladies, attention to these factors provides benefits ranging from simple feelings of well-being to enhanced athletic performance and resistance to disease.

While I have spent the past 25 years practicing medicine and exploring the frontiers of nutritional biochemistry, bringing innovative approaches to the day-to-day care of patients with challenging disorders, the fundamental and powerfully effective role of spirituality as part of a treatment regimen eluded me—until now.

■ ■ ■

It is now clear that ancient beliefs, coupled with modern beneficial physical and mental practices, may be the most powerful medicine of all—the way to power up your brain to seek, and attain, humanity's quest: enlightenment.

ENDNOTES

Introduction

1. Dan Buettner, *The Blue Zones: Lessons for Living Longer from the People Who've Lived the Longest* (Washington, DC: National Geographic, 2008).

Chapter 1: The Neuroscience of Enlightenment

1. Marcel Griaule (1898–1956), *The Pale Fox* (1965), translated from the French by Stephen C. Infantino (Chino Valley, AZ: Continuum Foundation, 1986).

2. Stuart R. Hameroff, *Ultimate Computing: Biomolecular Consciousness and Nanotechnology* (New York: Elsevier, 1987); Stuart R. Hameroff, Alfred W. Kaszniak, and Alwyn Scott (eds.), *Toward a Science of Consciousness* (Cambridge: MIT Press, 1996).

3. Jack A. Tuszynski, *The Emerging Physics of Consciousness* (New York: Springer, 2006).

4. His Holiness the Dalai Lama, *Becoming Enlightened* (New York: Atria Books, 2009), 88.

5. Ibid, 217.

Chapter 2: The Powerful Mind

1. W. Edward Craighead and Charles B. Nemeroff, *The Corsini Encyclopedia of Psychology and Behavioral Science*, vol. 3 (New York: John Wiley & Sons, 2001), 1212.

2. Darold A. Treffert, *Extraordinary People*, Backinprint.com, 2006.

Chapter 3: The Evolution of the Brain and the Mind

1. Deuteronomy 2:20, King James version.

Chapter 4: Mitochondria and the Feminine Life Force

1. To make a scientific distinction: Cells also have the ability to utilize other chemical pathways to produce ATP when oxygen is not present. However, this process, known as anaerobic metabolism, is only 1/18 as efficient as oxidative metabolism.

2. In a strict scientific sense, the term *free radicals* refers not only to reactive oxygen species, or ROS, but also to a similarly reactive family of radicals called reactive nitrogen species (RNS), but for purposes of simplification we use the term *free radicals* to refer to reactive oxygen species, which has become the norm in nonscientific publications.

3. Nick Lane, *Power, Sex, Suicide: Mitochondria and the Meaning of Life* (New York: Oxford University Press, 2005), p. 189.

4. J. F. R. Kerr, A. H. Wyllie, and A. R. Currie, "Apoptosis: A Basic Biological Phenomenon with Wide-Ranging Implications in Tissue Kinetics," *British Journal of Cancer* 26, no. 4 (August 1972): 239–57.

5. D. Harman, "Aging: A Theory Based on Free Radical and Radiation Chemistry," *Journal of Gerontology* 11, no. 3 (1956): 298–300.

6. See Lynn Margulis, *Symbiosis in Cell Evolution*, 2nd ed. (New York: W. H. Freeman, 1992).

Chapter 5: Neural Networks and Habits of the Mind

1. R. C. Kessler et al., "Posttraumatic Stress Disorder in the National Comorbidity Study," *Archives of General Psychiatry* 52, no. 12 (December 1995): 1048–60.

2. Ibid.

3. Julio F. Peres et al., "Cerebral Blood Flow Changes during Retrieval of Traumatic Memories before and after Psychotherapy: A SPECT Study," *Psychological Medicine* 37(October 2007): 1481–1491.

4. James Hillman, in the Preface to *The Logos of the Soul,* by Evangelos Christou (New York: Spring Publications, 2007): 8.

Chapter 6: How Stress Harms the Brain

1. Joan Stephenson, "Exposure to Home Pesticides Linked to Parkinson Disease," *Journal of the American Medical Association* 283, no. 23 (June 21, 2000): 3055–56.

2. "First BPA Detection in U.S. Infant Cord Blood," Environmental Working Group Press Release, December 2, 2009.

3. E. Dias-Ferreira et al., "Chronic Stress Causes Frontostriatal Reorganization and Affects Decision-Making," *Science* 325, no. 5940 (July 31, 2009): 621–25.

4. Robert M. Sapolsky quoted in Natalie Angier, "Brain is a Co-Conspirator in a Vicious Stress Loop," *New York Times,* August 17, 2009, http://www.nytimes.com/2009/08/18/science/18angier.html.

5. Robert M. Sapolsky, *Stress, the Aging Brain, and the Mechanisms of Neuron Death* (Cambridge: MIT Press, 1992), 327.

Chapter 7: The Gift of Neuroplasticity

1. See Begley, *Train Your Mind, Change Your Brain,* 158.

2. Ibid., 159.

3. Joe Dispenza, *Evolve Your Brain: The Science of Changing Your Mind* (Deerfield Beach, FL: HCI Books, 2007), 193–94.

4. Sharon Begley, "How Thinking Can Change the Brain," *Wall Street Journal,* January 19, 2007, http://online.wsj.com/ article/SB116915058061980596.html.

5. Alvaro Pascual-Leone et al., "The Plastic Human Brain Cortex," *Annual Review of Neuroscience* 28 (July 2005): 377–401.

6. Dispenza, *Evolve Your Brain,* 193.

7. See Begley, *Train Your Mind, Change Your Brain,* 152.

8. Jeffrey M. Schwartz and Sharon Begley, *The Mind and the Brain: Neuroplasticity and the Power of Mental Force* (New York: HarperCollins, 2003), 17–18.

9. Andrew Newberg and Mark Robert Waldman, *How God Changes Your Brain: Breakthrough Findings from a Leading Neuroscientist* (New York: Ballantine Books, 2009), 19–20.

10. Ibid., 124.

Chapter 8: Neurogenesis: Growing New Brain Cells

1. Begley, *Train Your Mind, Change Your Brain,* 65.

2. His Holiness the Dalai Lama, "Foreword," ibid., vii–viii.

3. Nicola Lautenschlager et al., "Effect of Physical Activity on Cognitive Function in Older Adults at Risk for Alzheimer's Disease," *Journal of the American Medical Association* 300, no. 9 (September 3, 2008):1027–37.

4. Jennifer Weuve et al., "Physical Activity, Including Walking, and Cognitive Function in Older Women," *Journal of the American Medical Association* 292, no. 12 (September 22, 2004):1454–61.

5. A. V. Witte et al., "Caloric Restriction Improves Memory in Elderly Humans," *Proceedings of the National Academy of Science* 106, no. 4 (January 27, 2009): 1255–60.

6. Mark P. Mattson et al., "Prophylactic Activation of Neuroprotective Stress Response Pathways by Dietary and Behavioral Manipulations," *NeuroRx* 1, no. 1 (January 2004): 112.

7. Ibid., 113.

8. Yakir Kaufman et al., "Cognitive Decline in Alzheimer Disease: Impact of Spirituality, Religiosity, and QOL," *Neurology* 68 (May 2007): 1509–14.

9. Karin Yurko-Mauro et al., "Results of the MIDAS Trial: Effects of Docosahexaenoic Acid on Physiological and Safety Parameters in Age-Related Cognitive Decline," *Alzheimer's & Dementia* 5, issue 4 (July 2009): 84.

Chapter 9: Three Conditions You Don't Want to Have

1. William R. Markesbery and Mark A. Lovell, "Damage to Lipids, Proteins, DNA, and RNA in Mild Cognitive Impairment," *Archives of Neurology* 64, no. 7 (July 2007): 954–56.

2. Ibid., 955.

3. Ling Gao et al., "Novel *n*-3 Fatty Acid Oxidation Products Activate Nrf2 by Destabilizing the Association between Keap1 and Cullin3," *Journal of Biological Chemistry* 282 (January 26, 2007): 2536.

4. M.R. Vargas et al., "Increased Glutathione Biosynthesis by Nrf2 Activation in Astrocytes Prevents p75NTR-dependent Motor Neuron Apoptosis," *Journal of Neurochemistry* 97, no. 3 (May 2006): 687–96.

5. Walter F. Stewart et al., "Risk of Alzheimer's Disease and Duration of NSAID Use," *Neurology* 48 (March 1997): 626–32; Honglei Chen et al., "Nonsteroidal Anti-inflammatory Drugs and the Risk of Parkinson's Disease," *Archives of Neurology* 60, no. 8 (August 2003): 1059–64.

6. A. Cagnin et al., "In-Vivo Measurement of Activated Microglia in Dementia," *Lancet* 358 (August 11, 2001): 461– 67.

7. Narayanan Venkatesan et al., "Curcumin Prevents Adriamycin Nephrotoxicity in Rats," *British Journal of Phramacology* 129, no. 2 (January 2000): 231–34.

8. T. L. Perry et al., "Parkinson's Disease: A Disorder Due to Nigral Glutathione Deficiency?" *Neuroscience Letters* 33, no. 3 (December 1982): 305–10.

9. D. Perlmutter and D. Townsend, "Parkinson's Disease: New Perspectives," *Townsend Letter for Doctors and Patients* (January 1997): 48–50.

Chapter 10: Cutting-Edge Therapies for Enhanced Energy Production

1. Personal communication, Dr. Richard Neubauer, December 20, 2006.

2. Glutathione available from Wellness Pharmacy, 3401 Independence Drive, Suite 231, Birmingham, AL 35209; (800) 227-2627

3. G. Sechi et al., "Reduced Intravenous Glutathione in the Treatment of Early Parkinson's Disease," *Progress in Neuro-Psychopharmacology and Biological Psychiatry* 20, no. 7 (October 1996): 1159–70.

4. Christopher A, Shaw (ed.), *Glutathione in the Nervous System* (Boca Raton, FL: CRC Press, 1998), 4.

5. L. Ye et al., "Quantitative Determination of Dithiocarbamates in Human Plasma, Serum, Erythrocytes and Urine: Pharmaco-kinetics of Broccoli Sprout Isothiocyanates in Humans," *International Journal of Clinical Chemistry* 316, nos. 1–2 (February 2002): 43–53.

Chapter 11: The Shaman's Gift

1. Calvin C. Clawson, *Mathematical Sorcery: Revealing the Secrets of Numbers* (New York: Basic Books, 2001), 10.

Chapter 12: Priming Your Brain for Enlightenment

1. William H. Calvin, *A Brain for All Seasons: Human Evolution and Abrupt Climate Change* (Chicago: University of Chicago Press, 2002), 307.

2. G. F. Cahill, Jr., and R. L. Veech, "Ketoacids? Good Medicine?" *Transactions of the American Clinical and Climatological Association* 114 (2003): 149.

3. M. A. Reger et al., "Effects of Beta-hydroxybutyrate on Cognition in Memory-impaired Adults," *Neurobiology of Aging* 25, no. 3 (March 2004): 311–14.

4. See http://www.treeoflife.nu/media-library/ articles-videos-more/why-fast/.

5. Paramahansa Yogananda, *Man's Eternal Quest: Collected Talks and Essays,* vol. 1 (Los Angeles: Self-Realization Fellowship, 1982), 107.

6. Thomas Ryan, CSP, *The Sacred Art of Fasting: Preparing to Practice* (Woodstock, VT: SkyLight Paths Publishing, 2005), 163.

7. N. T. Lautenschlager et al., "Effect of Physical Activity on Cognitive Function in Older Adults at Risk for Alzheimer Disease," *Journal of the American Medical Association* 300, no. 9 (September 3, 2008): 1027–37.

8. J. Weuve et al., "Physical Activity, Including Walking, and Cognitive Function in Older Women," *Journal of the American Medical Association* 292, no. 12 (September 2004): 1454–61.

9. R. D. Abbott et al., "Walking and Dementia in Physically Capable Elderly Men," *Journal of the American Medical Association* 292, no. 12 (September 2004): 1447–53.

Chapter 13: Shamanic Exercises

1. E. Epel et al., "Can Meditation Slow Rate of Cellular Aging? Cognitive Stress, Mindfulness, and Telomeres," *Annals of the New York Academy of Sciences* 1172 (August 2009): 34–53.

2. Poetic rendering of the Yoga Sutras of Patanjali, 1.32, by Alberto Villoldo, in *Yoga, Power, and Spirit: Patanjali the Shaman* (New York: Hay House, 2007), 27.

Chapter 14: The Power Up Your Brain Program

1. Celiac Disease Awareness Campaign of the National Institutes of Health, "Provider Points: Testing for Celiac Disease," http://digestive.niddk.nih.gov/ddiseases/pubs/celiactesting/ Celiac_Testing_CDAC_PP.pdf.

2. Your doctor can perform this test by contacting Genova Diagnostics at (800) 522-4762 or at www.genovadiagnostics.com.

3. "Moderate Drinking Can Reduce Risks Of Alzheimer's Dementia And Cognitive Decline, Analysis Suggests," *Science Daily,* December 31, 2008, http://www.sciencedaily.com/releases/2008/12/081229200750.htm.

Chapter 15: Searching for Your Soul

1. Alberto Villoldo and Erik Jendresen, *Dance of the Four Winds: Secrets of the Inca Medicine Wheel* (Rochester, VT: Destiny Books, 1994), 10.

ACKNOWLEDGMENTS

We gratefully acknowledge Robert Weir and Nancy Peske, who proved overwhelmingly successful in meeting the challenge of melding two seemingly disparate voices into a cohesive whole. We extend our sincere gratitude to the Hay House team including Patty Gift, whose vision and insight have sustained this project from its inception; and Laura Koch for her spot-on commentary and editorial prowess; as well as Reid Tracy, Richelle Zizian, Johanne Mahaffey, Sally Mason, and Christy Salinas.

ABOUT THE
AUTHORS

David Perlmutter, M.D., F.A.C.N., is a board-certified neurologist and fellow of the American College of Nutrition. He serves as medical director of the Perlmutter Health Center and the Perlmutter Hyperbaric Center in Naples, Florida, and is also an adjunct instructor at the Institute for Functional Medicine.

Dr. Perlmutter is recognized internationally as a leader in the field of nutritional influences in neurological disorders. In 2002, he was awarded the Linus Pauling Award for his work in innovative approaches to neurological disorders, and in the same year he received the Denham Harman Award for his work in advancing the understanding of free radical biochemistry in neurological diseases. He also received the 2006 National Nutritional Foods Association Clinician of the Year Award and the 2010 Humanitarian of the Year Award from the American College of Nutrition.

Dr. Perlmutter has contributed extensively to the world of medical literature with publications in numerous journals. He is also the author of four books: *BrainRecovery.com, The Better Brain Book, LifeGuide: Your Guide to a Longer and Healthier Life,* and *Raise a Smarter Child by Kindergarten.*

Dr. Perlmutter has been interviewed on many nationally syndicated radio and television programs including *20/20, The Faith Daniels Program, Larry King Live,* CNN, Fox News, *Fox & Friends,* the *Today* show, *The Oprah Winfrey Show,* and CBS's *The Early Show.*

Website: **www.DrPerlmutter.com**

Alberto Villoldo, Ph.D., has trained as a psychologist and medical anthropologist, and has studied the healing practices of the Amazon and the Andean shamans for more than 25 years. While an adjunct professor San Francisco State University, he founded the Biological Self-Regulation Laboratory to study how the mind creates psychosomatic health and disease. Convinced that the mind could create health, he left his laboratory and traveled to the Amazon to work with the medicine men and women of the rainforest and learn their healing methods and mythology.

Dr. Villoldo directs The Four Winds Society, where he trains individuals in the U.S. and Europe in the practice of shamanic energy medicine. He is the founder of the Healing the Light Body School, which has campuses in New York, California, Park City, Australia, the UK, Sweden, Holland, and Germany. He currently directs the Four Winds Society in the USA and the Center for Energy Medicine in Chile, where he investigates and practices the neuroscience of enlightenment.

Websites: **www.thefourwinds.com** and
www.PowerUpYourBrain.com

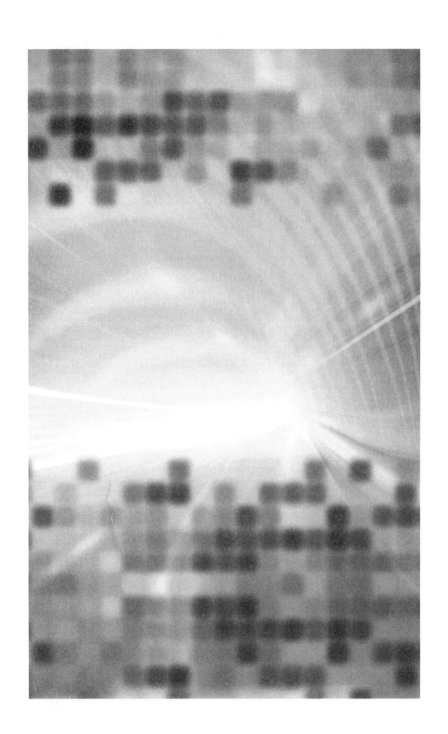

NOTES

NOTES

NOTES

NOTES

NOTES

NOTES

NOTES

NOTES

NOTES

NOTES

Hay House Titles of Related Interest

YOU CAN HEAL YOUR LIFE, the movie,
starring Louise L. Hay & Friends
(available as a 1-DVD program and an expanded 2-DVD set)
Watch the trailer at: **www.LouiseHayMovie.com**

THE SHIFT, the movie,
starring Dr. Wayne W. Dyer
(available as a 1-DVD program and an expanded 2-DVD set)
Watch the trailer at: **www.DyerMovie.com**

■ ■ ■

THE BIOLOGY OF BELIEF: Unleashing the Power of Consciousness, Matter & Miracles, by Bruce H. Lipton, Ph.D.

COURAGEOUS DREAMING: How Shamans Dream the World into Being, by Alberto Villoldo, Ph.D.

ILLUMINATION: The Shaman's Way of Healing,
by Alberto Villoldo, Ph.D.

THE SPONTANEOUS HEALING OF BELIEF: Shattering the Paradigm of False Limits, by Gregg Braden

All of the above are available at your local bookstore,
or may be ordered by contacting Hay House (see next page).

■ ■ ■